Sociological and Spiritual Aspects of Palliative Care in Ireland

Understandings of a "Good Death"

SOCIOLOGICAL AND SPIRITUAL ASPECTS OF PALLIATIVE CARE IN IRELAND

Understandings of a "Good Death"

Una MacConville

With a Foreword by
Allan Kellehear

The Edwin Mellen Press
Lewiston•Queenston•Lampeter

Library of Congress Cataloging-in-Publication Data

MacConville, Una.
Sociological and spiritual aspects of palliative care in Ireland : understandings of a "good death" / Una MacConville ; with a foreword by Allan Kellehear.
p. cm.
Includes bibliographical references and index.
ISBN-13: 978-0-7734-1570-6 (hardcover)
ISBN-10: 0-7734-1570-X (hardcover)
1. Death--Social aspects--Ireland. 2. Palliative treatment--Social aspects--Ireland. 3. Hospice care--Social aspects--Ireland. 4. Hospice care--Religious aspects--Catholic Church. I. Title.
HQ1073.5.I73M33 2011
362.17'5088282417--dc23
2011016078

hors série.

A CIP catalog record for this book is available from the British Library.

Front cover: *Coming to and going from III* © Catherine MacConville (2008) painting

The Edwin Mellen Press
Box 450
Lewiston, New York
USA 14092-0450

The Edwin Mellen Press
Box 67
Queenston, Ontario
CANADA L0S 1L0

The Edwin Mellen Press, Ltd.
Lampeter, Ceredigion, Wales
UNITED KINGDOM SA48 8LT

Printed in the United States of America

For Kathleen and Dermot

TABLE OF CONTENTS

FOREWORD

How are we to understand how the complex array of social, psychological, physical and spiritual intricacies and intimacies that influences the dying person, and the dying body, at the end of life? How are health services to address this complexity of dying sensitively, in social and culture-specific ways that make sense to the dying person, their families and communities? Religious meanings are multiple in modern affluent societies, and often sit alongside secular and agnostic views about the fate of the person after death. Work occupation, citizenship or wealth no longer predicts with any confidence the social values, attitudes and preferences of many people today. And although we have become accustomed to the habit of re-drawing our global maps to take into account the emerging new regimes, nations and international alliances, the maps of death, dying and care are in their infancy. These 'maps' remain partial and poorly explored — they are often uncertain, debatable and subject to much anxiety. MacConville provides us with the first powerful and explicit attempt to describe a modern 'map' of dying and its care.

In this study, from inside a palliative care services approach, MacConville identifies two important physical and social 'countries' — the dying person-in-community and the dying person-in-professional care. In the former, the dying person and family experience professional carers as guests or as visitors; and in the other the dying person in professional environs is the visitor and guest. These situations, in gross outline, show us an immediate set of similarities but also contrasts, of convergence and collision. In close-up detail, MacConville's maps of care show us what some map-makers describe as 'fractals' — those parts of coast and crag that fail to show up on major relief maps because they are too infinite and idiosyncratic in detail. These fractals need finer examination by the unwary traveller. From these nuanced observations a map of coasts or dying is transformed for the experienced eye. This is the promise and the originality of MacConville's landmark work. MacConville provides us with a new way of viewing both dying and its care while at the same time as offering a new theoretical framework for charting Shakespeare's—and our—'undiscovered country'. This is a worthy, challenging and pioneering contribution.

Professor Allan Kellehear

Centre for Death & Society, University of Bath, UK

PREFACE

This book explores understandings of a 'good death' and the spiritual dimension of care in an Irish palliative care setting. It sets out to fill some of what Norbert Elias observed as 'blank areas on the social map of death and dying'. Elias was writing in the early 1980s, and since that time there has been a huge increase in interest and research about death and dying. Notwithstanding this, there are still many blank areas on a social map of death and dying and especially so in Ireland, where little research has been conducted.

A 'GOOD DEATH'

A 'good death' is an almost universal concept. It is usually an attempt to exert some level of control over the biological event of death; the type of control and the means of exercising it change over time and across cultures. Contemporary representations of a 'good death' demonstrate that a 'good death' is not fixed and can be negotiated. For example, Bradbury (1999, 144) has asserted that representations of 'good' and 'bad' deaths are 'culturally prescribed ways of viewing death which serve to delineate the social order'.

Palliative care is concerned with the relief of symptoms and with optimising the psychological, social and spiritual well-being of patients whose disease is no longer responsive to curative treatment. A central tenet of palliative care is the facilitation of a 'good death'; however, the definition of this is not always clear. Research (such as Payne and Langley-Evans 1996; Dekkers *et al.* 2002) has shown that while patients, family and staff share some views about what a 'good death' might entail, a 'good death' is also a highly individual experience. Spiritual care is a further element of a 'good death' and is an important dimension of palliative care. However, this too can be somewhat problematic, owing to a lack of a shared definition.

Underlying the concept of a 'good death' and the spiritual dimension of palliative care is a distinction between the individual and the social experience of death and dying. This book documents an ethnographic study that explored the views of doctors, nurses, chaplains, social workers, administration and household staff in an Irish hospice about these aspects. Themes of mapping and social space have assisted in making explicit these distinctions and the specific cultural, historical and political contexts in which both the individual and the social aspects of death and dying are located.

SOCIAL MAPS

Maps, social or otherwise, vary in their size and focus. Maps that represent large physical areas are generally small in scale, useful for an overview when travelling from one part of a country to another. These types of maps provide the larger picture, the quickest or most direct route to follow and the broad outline of topographical features: cities, mountains, rivers and so on. A closer and more detailed picture is revealed in maps of a different scale; the large-scale six-inch maps, or pathfinder maps, can disclose far more. The detail provided by these maps shows more clearly the multi-layered nature of the physical and social worlds, shaped by interactions in the past and in the present. For example, maps of this scale can not only provide the detail of topographical features such as mountains and rivers but, can also show the presence of ancient monuments, medieval settlements and abandoned industrial sites in addition to present-day structures and institutions.

Cartography and social space are a central focus of this study. 'Mapping' and the creation of 'maps' have been developed and used as an organising principle, a methodological approach to understanding relationships within palliative care that shape and influence perceptions of a 'good death' and spiritual care and, ultimately, as a way of distinguishing between uniquely individual aspects and the shared social experience of death and dying.

The relationships between physical and social worlds are apparent on maps of sufficient scale. Relationships, between patients, family members and professional staff, are a dominant theme of this study. These dynamics, clearly revealed in the actual physical space occupied by the participants within their social and political contexts and over time, set in motion what Lefebvre considers a 'specific dialectic' in which 'a unity transpires between levels which analysis keeps separate from one another' (1991, 85). I found clear differences in the relationships between health care professionals and patients and their families according to the location of care. For instance, palliative care professionals are 'visitors' in the homes of patients, while patients become 'visitors' in the in-patient unit of the hospice. Examining these relationships in relation to place enabled the manners of engagement of these relationships to be more clearly understood.

Cartography also influenced the methodology of the study—one of exploration and map-making and an *emic* framework—which builds on the narrative of the participants without attempting to steer it into any pre-formed categories. This approach has been advocated by Corr *et al.*, who suggest that an *etic* framework—in which the culture is slotted into the visitor's linguistic and conceptual categories—has been the hallmark of most theories of dying (1999, 250).

Within an *emic* framework, the role of the researcher can more clearly be seen as that of a visitor in the social world of the participants and in the hospice. Viewing the role of the researcher in this way highlighted the dynamics involved in entering into other social worlds—that of the hospice and the participants—and the responsibilities or ethical considerations that this entails. The degree to which the researcher can become assimilated into these worlds, becoming part of the family and less of a visitor, depends on the degree of trust and intimacy that develops and is an important aspect of qualitative research.

The application of a cartographic approach also helped to clarify the degree to which the uniquely individual aspect of death and dying can be understood. An analogy has been drawn between the physical landscape and the social worlds of patients and family members in order to make explicit how much or how little is known or can be known or even should be known.

The analogy between the physical and social worlds has an explanatory value beyond the current subject-matter of a 'good death' and spiritual care. The unique aspect of any individual experience, the part that cannot be known by another, has been likened to 'fractals' on the coastal landscape. This is a mathematical concept, adapted by cartographer Tim Robinson, to describe the infinite and ultimately unmappable elements of the landscape. In relation to this study what can be 'mapped' are the intersections, that part of the individual experience that intersects with the social world, comprised of multiple social actors and institutions, each in relationship with each other. Just as the six-inch map can reveal the multi-layered nature of the interaction between the physical and social worlds over time, social maps can convey the historical, political and social contexts in which social actors and institutions are located.

This study also can be considered as a social map, albeit a social map that still contains many blank areas. Section 1 of this book is entitled 'The known world' and contains three chapters. The first chapter focuses on what is already known about a 'good death', spiritual care, and the development of palliative care in locations other than Ireland. Chapter 2 presents the social and historical context for the research—Ireland, like any other cultural setting, has a cultural and historical specificity that shapes definitions of a 'good death' and spiritual care. Chapter 3 outlines the methodology of the research—the means of exploration.

Section 2 can be considered as a series of 'sketch-maps'. Chapters 4, 5 and 6 are largely descriptive and set out the social landscape. They are akin to the landscape sketches of early explorers and move from broad brush strokes depicting the culture of palliative care to the organisational structures and relationships, and how these change according to the location of care. Chapters 7 and 8 present the ways in which spiritual care and a 'good death' were perceived and interpreted within the hospice.

The final section can be considered as the key to these sketches or 'maps' and provides the 'legend' for understanding the topography depicted in the previous chapters. It pulls together the emergent themes of the research and discusses Elias's figurational approach as an aid to understanding the relationships both with and between individuals and institutions. Chapters 9 and 10 explore how these relationships have been shaped by the past, how they are conducted in the present and the importance of making explicit the dynamics present in these relationships.

ACKNOWLEDGEMENTS

Many people and institutions have assisted and supported me in undertaking this research and in bringing the results to published form. Firstly I would like to extend my gratitude and appreciation to all those who took part in this study; without their commitment, interest and willingness to share their experiences this study could not have been undertaken. I would also like to thank Professor Glennys Howarth for her unwavering support and encouragement over the years and her belief in social maps, especially when I began to doubt them myself.

I would further like to thank the University of Bath and the Economic and Social Research Council for financial scholarships that enabled me to undertake this research, and in particular to express my gratitude to Dr Mark Baldwin and Dr Nick Gould, of the University of Bath, for their support and guidance. My thanks are also due to Professor Allan Kellehear for generously providing the foreword for this book and to Tim Robinson for his kind permission to reproduce illustrations from his published work.

Undertaking this research and the preparation for publication have taken a number of years and I would like to thank my family and friends, whose support and encouragement have helped me bring this to completion. In particular, I would like to thank my husband, Nick Maxwell, and my children Aoife, Ruaidhrí and Meadhbh for their support, patience and understanding.

SECTION 1
THE KNOWN WORLD

INTRODUCTION

The title of this section is 'The known world'. In keeping with the cartographic approach adopted, this section presents what is already known and present in the literature regarding a 'good death', spiritual care and the development of palliative care for the care of the dying. It also presents, in Chapter 2, the social and political contexts of care for the dying in Ireland. Chapter 3 presents the methodology of the research, or, in cartographic terms, the 'means of exploration' for filling in the blank areas on the social map that Elias has identified.

Birth and death are the two inescapable facts of human existence. At birth individuals arrive into the known and ordered social world, however that is constituted. In death, individuals leave this social world, moving from the known to the unknown. In nearly all cultures stories have been told of travel to another world in which mortals pass through the gates of death and return with messages for the living (Zaleski 1987), but the truth of these stories can only be attested by those who do not return.

Elias (1985) states that death is a problem of the living; dead people have no problems. Human beings are alone in finding death a problem, Elias argues, because only they know that they will die; they can anticipate their end and are aware that it can come at any time, and therefore there is a need to take special precautions—as individuals and as groups—to protect themselves against the danger of annihilation (*op. cit.*, 4).

Death is a journey into the unknown which belongs only to the individual who embarks on it, but the manner of embarkation and the parting from friends and family is a social experience and takes place within an existing social order. Elias (*op. cit.*, 1) has suggested that it is our task to 'make the end, the parting from human beings, when it comes, as easy and as pleasant as possible, for others as well as ourselves'. This poses a question of how this might be accomplished. A 'good death' is about the manner of parting and the tasks that need to be accomplished in order to make that as easy and as pleasant as possible. How these tasks are defined and accomplished changes over time and across cultures.

Beliefs in an afterlife, another social world, are also almost universal to all cultures. These beliefs represent, according to Elias, the human endeavour to come to terms with the finiteness of life and have been mythologised through ideas of an afterlife such as Valhalla or Hades, Heaven or Hell. Whatever the nature of these beliefs and however an afterlife is constituted, preparation for it is also part of a 'good death'; the form of preparation is shaped by individual beliefs and values but also by the culture of the social world in which the individual resides.

CHAPTER 1
The manner of parting

This chapter is a consideration of the variety of ways in which partings are made and understood and the attempts to restore or minimise the disorder that may ensue or to 'make them as easy as possible'. Historical and contemporary accounts of parting are considered, as are preparations for an afterlife, and the way in which these are shaped by the cultural social order in which death occurs is reviewed. The social order of palliative care and how this model of health care has developed and shaped the manner of parting is also considered.

A 'good death'

A 'good death' is about the manner of parting and the tasks that need to be accomplished in order to make that as easy and as pleasant as possible, as Elias has stated. How this is done changes over time and across cultures and is conceptualised in ideas about 'good' and 'bad' deaths.

Concepts of 'good' and 'bad' deaths are present in most cultures. Bloch and Parry have discussed the constitution of 'good' and 'bad' deaths within the anthropological record and argue that the drive to 'determine the time and place of death and the dissociation of social death from bodily death represents an attempt to control the unpredictable nature of biological death and dramatise the victory of order over biology' (1982, 15). In this sense a 'good death' is one that suggests some level of control over the biological event, while 'bad' deaths are those which demonstrate the absence of control.

Control over death or the manner of death is linked by Bloch and Parry with the regenerative power of death in maintaining order, lineage and societal continuance. 'Bad' deaths, such as those caused by accident or suicide, preclude the chance of regeneration and also make the task of imposing order on potential disorder more difficult. Bradbury (1999), in developing the arguments of Bloch and Parry in contemporary western societies, states that there is a considerable degree of negotiation, and disagreement, over what constitutes a 'good' or a 'bad' death. For instance, not all suicides are viewed negatively—the idea of negatively sanctioned suicide and positively sanctioned suicide was first considered by Durkheim (1952). A social group engaged in war may portray the death of young healthy men as a 'good death', although how these deaths are represented is dependent upon particular viewpoints; for example, the death of a hunger-striker can be viewed differently according to political viewpoints. A 'good death' is therefore as much about a 'good life', a justification for existing social behaviour and order, as about the manner of parting. Representations of 'good' and 'bad' deaths are, according to Bradbury (1999, 144), 'culturally prescribed ways of viewing death which serve to delineate the social order'.

Historical representations of a 'good death'

Representations of a 'good death' reflect the cultures of the societies in which they are located. *Ars moriendi*, 'the art of dying', was a body of Christian devotional literature introduced in Europe in the fourteenth and fifteenth centuries. It included a variety of reflections on the themes of death and dying and represented an appropriation by the laity of a tradition of monastic penitential practices (Bartley 2001). This happened at a time, according to Bartley, of generalised anxiety arising from the religious and economic crises of the period. Works such as William Caxton's *Arte and Crafte to know well to dye* (1490) have been likened by Morgan (1999, 128) to 'distance learning packs' for those who were dying, but also for those who might organise the deathbed. They were essentially manuals on how people ought to die rather than revealing how they did actually die (from Aston 1994). The emphasis in these texts was primarily on the doctrines concerning the salvation of the soul and the condition of the dying person's soul, although they included practical management of the deathbed.

In an account of deathbed scenes in England in the Early Modern period (1558–1660) Gittings (1999) states that, in line with Protestant theology, depictions of deathbeds concentrated on worldly rather than on spiritual matters. One's earthly possessions were required to be in good order, although it was also considered important for the dying person to be at peace with God and with his or her fellow men. Particular importance was placed on the right speeches before death and on being conscious at death.

The Victorian era saw a return to the medieval tradition of *ars moriendi*, as religion played a powerful role in the lives of most middle- and upper-class Victorians (Jalland 1999). The Victorian 'good death' required 'piety and lifelong preparation'. It should also

> *'take place in a good Christian home, surrounded by loving and supportive family, with the dying person making explicit farewells to family members, comforted by the assurance of future family reunions in Heaven' (ibid., 233).*

Catholic 'good deaths'

In cultures such as Catholic Spain, the presence of certain members of the family and close friends was encouraged, but wives, children, fathers and mothers were not 'because those do not help in avoiding temptations, even more, with their great passion in considering what they are losing, they even increase the agony' (Fernández-Shaw Toda 1997). In their place,

> *'those companions should be two or three good friends, catholic, discrete and charitable, in order to help when he is still lucid to prepare himself for dying, advise him to write a testament and get ready to receive his last sacraments' (from* Agonía del tránsito de la muerte— *'Agony of the passing of death'* —written in 1537 and quoted by Fernández-Shaw Toda).

The presence of a priest or priests is important for a Catholic 'good death'; an account by Ariès (1994, 7) of a death in nineteenth-century rural France emphasises the role of the priest at the deathbed and the role of the community in caring for the dying. Accounts of death customs in Ireland, based on a questionnaire circulated by the Department of Folklore at University College Dublin in 1976, reflect a similar picture.

These accounts show general attitudes towards the dying (Lysaght 1995, 27) in which the family and community, as well as the priest, play a large part. They reveal a common picture of dying in familiar surroundings, at home, in the presence of family and friends, and having received the consolation of one's religion.

Attending to temporal matters such as disputes or outstanding debts was considered important, 'in order to lessen the load on the soul going before God' (Lysaght 1995, 33). The presence of the priest at the bedside of the dying person, in order to administer the Last Sacraments, was also important; 'it was the priest who was always sent for before the doctor in case the speech might leave him and he would not be able to make a full confession' (*op. cit.*, 34). Lysaght states that the administration of the Last Sacraments and the devotional atmosphere in the sickroom were felt to bring peace and resignation to the dying person for the journey towards death. It also imparted peace, comfort and calmness to the bystanders—the family and community—'to whom the spiritual as well as the physical care of the dying person reverted after the priest has left, if the person was still alive' (*op. cit.*, 39).

Contemporary representations of a 'good death'

Kellehear (1990, 57) states that the contemporary 'good death' has become more complex as the social commitments and responsibilities of modern industrial people are now broader than the religious ones of the society of the *ars moriendi*. Walter (1994) has considered the broad social changes in death and dying over time and has focused on a movement from traditional to modern and toward neo-modern. Three aspects of these types of deaths—bodily context, social context and authority—are also considered.

The traditional form of a 'good death' was, according to Walter, characterised by infectious disease from which people died quickly, generally at home amongst their family and community and with a faith in religious authority. In contrast, the modern 'good death' is characterised by more people living to old age, and medical professionals increasingly manage death when it occurs. A splitting of the private and public spheres emerges; the feelings of the dying and the grieving are private and authority is vested in expertise, such as that of the medical staff (1994, 52). According to Walter, neo-modern deaths mean that terminal diagnosis of cancer and other life-threatening illnesses are made explicit and, with improved medical treatment and care, people are living longer with incurable illnesses, leading to a prolonged and conscious dying trajectory. Changes in the split between private and public have, according to Walter, led to private experience being made public and that now the ultimate authority is the self (*op. cit.*, 54).

Bradbury (1999) presents three representations of a 'good death'—a 'sacred good death', a 'medical good death' and a 'natural good death'—which emerged from her ethnographic research amongst death-workers (hospital chaplain, a parish priest, hospital nurses, patients' affairs officer, police officers, coroners and so on) and widows in England. Bradbury found, in line with other studies (such as Kellehear 1990), a number of factors that contributed to a 'good death': awareness of the dying period, preparation for the death, pain control, the presence of a spouse and/or family at the death, and for many people in the study dying at home was important.

Nevertheless, within the representations that Bradbury presents there are often quite paradoxical ideas. Bradbury states that in her study she found several examples of deaths considered as 'natural' that were 'an extraordinary and often contradictory jumble' (1999, 152). Some deaths occurred as a result of accidents or at least unexpectedly. These were considered as 'natural' in part because they seemed to 'fit' with the life of the deceased; for instance, for some it was a 'good death' because there was no protracted period of illness, which would have been unacceptable for the deceased. One respondent, whose husband died after several weeks of care at home, felt that the death acquired a 'naturalness' because of mutual preparation.

Other representations of a 'good death' in Bradbury's study also contain a mix of traditional and modern aspects. The deathbed scene seemed to play a central role in a 'sacred good death'. The women in Bradbury's study spoke about the awareness-consciousness of their dying husbands, the presence of family and friends, and even the general setting such as music and candles, and these aspects seem to draw on traditional images of dying the 'good death'. At the same time these good deaths are modern events in which medical science plays a central role (*op. cit.*, 147).

One particular account highlights that a 'good death' can be viewed from a number of perspectives. One widow in the study described the death of her husband as 'perfect': he died surrounded by his family, at home, they played a recording of his favourite sonata and opened a bottle of champagne to celebrate his well-lived life (*op. cit.*, 147). According to this widow, the deathbed scene was 'orchestrated' by her local hospital's terminal support team, who administered high levels of opiates. While this description may provide an idealised scene, this widow also described her husband's fight against death to the very last moments of his life 'as he thrashed and writhed about on the bed', suggesting a marked contrast between the idealised scene and the reality for the dying person.

A further representation in Bradbury's study is that of a 'medical good death'. Although not always the case, it would appear that this category related to sudden or unexpected deaths in which all efforts were directed towards life-saving activities, whether successful or not. Bradbury maintains that the appearance of medical intervention was enough to ensure a 'good death', as the comments from one doctor in her research show: 'I mean, quite often, if you bring them in and they are obviously dead you will actually wait ten minutes so the relatives think you have done something' (*op. cit.*, 151). These comments suggest that the 'medical good death' may transform a potentially 'bad death' through the apparent exercise of some level of control and expertise. The medical interventions in these cases, in contrast to the 'natural' death, are welcomed as they have a transformative function and represent a mechanism for control.

The medicalisation of death

Howarth (1996) argues that people have always desired control over death. Historically this was pursued through religious belief. In the contemporary western world, with the declining role of Christianity, science and technology have largely replaced faith as a means of making sense of mortality (1996, 13).

Jalland (1999, 242) maintains that by the end of the nineteenth century in England increased religious doubt and Evangelical decline, matched with a revised view of disease, combined to attribute the cause of death to particular diseases rather than to divine providence. Bradbury (1999) argues that during the eighteenth and nineteenth centuries representations of death changed along with medical innovations. Dying was a process that could increasingly be made painless through the application of powerful painkillers. The development of a secular climate of opinion changed not only the manner of a 'good death' but also its meaning. The 'good death' was no longer concerned with the fate of the soul; it was concerned with the character of the physical event (1999, 192). Bradbury also contends that the medical notion of a 'good death' remains the dominant representation and the hospital environment provides the optimal degree of control.

Hockey (1990) has argued that since the eighteenth century a view of death as part of the natural cycle of life was overtaken by a concern to control the process of dying with medical remedies; people began trying to negotiate with death. In this context Illich's (1977, 204) discussion of the iconography of death reflects the increasing importance of the doctor's interventionist role. As Illich relates, in the age of the Dance of Death (fourteenth–fifteenth century) the inclusion of the physician is rare and the skeleton makes the doctor the butt of his jokes. In the eighteenth century death seems to enjoy teasing the doctor about his diagnoses. With the development of 'clinical sickness and clinical death' the picture changes to the doctor interposing himself between death and the patient. After the First World War doctors are seen wrangling with the skeleton, and 'by 1930 a smiling white-coated man is rushing against a whimpering skeleton and crushing it like a fly with two volumes of Marle's Lexicon of Therapy' (Illich 1977, 204).

Elias (1985) has considered the changes in attitudes to death as part of long-term social processes, akin to other civilising social processes. Elias, writing in the early 1980s, commented that 'never before in the history of humanity have the dying been removed so hygienically behind the scenes of social life' (*op. cit.*, 23). Illich (1977, 210) argues that the medicalisation of society brought 'natural death' to an end and 'western man has lost the right to preside at his act of dying', and in its place the 'good death' has become that 'of the standard consumer of medical care .... [men] are stamped from birth as patients who need all kinds of treatment if they want to lead life the right way' (*op. cit.*, 202). In the context of medical science the 'natural' death is a bad death that took place without any kind of treatment, a domain of the disordered, unpredictable and uncontrolled (Hockey 1990).

It appears that, on the one hand, a death can be represented as 'natural' when there is medical intervention and, on the other hand, as 'natural' when it represents a break from what is increasingly seen as the 'overbearing and intrusive medical control of the dying' (Bradbury 1999, 154). De Beauvoir (1966, 106) has reflected, in relation to the death of her mother, that 'there is no such thing as a natural death; nothing that happens to man is ever natural'. The apparent contradiction between conceptualisations of 'natural' and the role of medical technology are certainly not straightforward (Seymour 1999). According to Seymour, accounts of lay respondents show a 'warp and weft effect of ideas drawn from a variety of sources and combined such that medical intervention during dying is portrayed as sometimes supportive of a "natural" way of dying and at other times in opposition to a "natural" way' (1999, 698).

This weaving of individual ideas about 'natural' and 'unnatural' is characteristic of what Walter (1994) considers neo-modern death, as already mentioned. Neo-modern death features the key characteristics of post-modernism—double coding, a mixing of traditional and modern elements to create a new form (from Jencks 1990, cited in Walter 1994) —and combines features of traditional and modern ways of death and dying. The natural death movement established in the early 1990s (Albery *et al.* 1993) was based loosely on the natural birth movement of the 1970s, which argued for the rights of women to give birth without unnecessary and intrusive medical interventions. The association with the natural birth movement links Illich's reference to being 'stamped as patients' from birth. In a departure from Illich's view of a medicalised society, however, the natural death movement seeks to redress the balance and, while not advocating that people die without any kind of pain relief or intervention, the dying are encouraged to take control of their dying and to reject a passive 'patient' role (Bradbury 1999, 155).

Negotiating a 'good death'

The representations of a 'good death' in Bradbury's study, already discussed, present often contradictory ideas and emphasise the degree to which 'good deaths' are managed and negotiated by social actors rather than being fixed. Interpretations are also not fixed in time, and meaning can be subject to a process of interpretation that can continue long after the experience of the event (Seymour 1999, 698). Williamson (1990, 121), in a study of attitudes to death and illness amongst older people in Aberdeen, has described how his respondents' attitudes to dying appear as '...historical strata laid down by a culture in motion', and how 'potentially paradoxical ideas about the role of nature, medicine, religion and self determination' are contextualised in order to represent particular values or experiences.

A study by Young and Cullen (1996), based on research in the East End of London, captures the ways in which a 'good death' is negotiated by individuals, families and professionals through a multitude of pathways—personal sensibilities, life experience, cultural expectations and restrictions and most of all, as the authors state, 'the significance of people's spirit—the quality that belongs to the whole personality and how that whole personality reacts to adversity' (*op. cit.*, 36).

Bradbury's (1999) study provides an insightful look at contemporary representations of death and captures the way in which these representations of a 'good death' are negotiated and managed by individuals and by professionals. Walter (1994) also provides a useful broad consideration of social change. Little research, however, has been undertaken to capture the cultural diversity of death and dying in contemporary Britain, which is a multi-cultural society. Bradbury does make reference to the difficulties experienced in negotiating a 'good death' for British Hindus within the institutional constraints of hospitals and hospices (citing Firth's 1996 study of British Hindu death in southern England). Walter suggests that within modern western societies, medicine has created a modern or neo-modern context for death but that this can coexist with more traditional social contexts (1994, 49), such as those within remote rural areas (Clark 1982), immigrant groups (Firth 1993; Kalish and Reynolds 1981) and the Irish of Belfast and Dublin (Prior 1989). While there appears to be scope for individual negotiation of whether a death is good or bad, it is also clear that this negotiation takes place within broad cultural scripts: a Catholic 'good death' may differ in some respects from a Protestant one, and the wealthy may have access to additional resources beyond the reach of many. Bradbury asserts that representations of 'good' and 'bad' deaths are 'culturally prescribed ways of viewing death which serve to delineate the social order'. Nevertheless, the means to negotiate a 'good death' are not necessarily evenly distributed.

Palliative care

The World Health Organisation has defined palliative care as the active, total care of patients whose disease is no longer responsive to curative treatment. Control of pain and symptoms and of psychological, social and spiritual problems is paramount. The goal of palliative care is the achievement of the best possible quality of life for patients and their families (WHO 1990). Underlying this WHO definition are the principles of palliative care—an emphasis on open awareness of death and dying and communication and the concept of 'total pain', which considers pain to be multidimensional (physical, psychological, social and spiritual). These will be discussed later in this chapter.

Quality of life is a difficult concept to define and measure; it has a usage across many disciplines—literature, philosophy, politics, health promotion, medicine and the social sciences (O'Boyle and Waldron 1997). The WHO Quality of Life (WHOQol) working party has provided the following definition of quality of life: 'Quality of life is defined as the individual's perception of their position in life in the context of the culture and value systems in which they live and in relation to their goals, expectations, standards and concerns. It is a broad ranging concept affected in a complex way by a person's physical health, psychological state, level of independence and their relationship to salient features in their environment' (*ibid.*,

S20). This definition underpins the development of the WHOQol core measure, specific editions of which are planned for various groups such as cancer patients (Szabo 1996).

The evolution of palliative care

Palliative care has developed from hospice care. Hospices, as places to care for the dying, have a long history and can be documented from the fourth century with the establishment by St Fabiola of a hospice for pilgrims staffed by religious orders. Medieval hospices were dedicated to the sick and dying and the Christian burial of the dead. In the nineteenth century (1836) Pastor Fliednor founded the first Protestant order of deaconesses at Kaiserworth, whose duties included the care of the dying. In 1842 Mme Ganier, a Roman Catholic widow, founded the hospice for the dying in France. The Irish Sisters of Charity opened a hospice in Dublin in 1879 and in London in 1904. In the US the first hospice was established in 1899 by Dominican nuns, a special order called 'the servants for the relief of incurable cancer', who opened six more hospices in the United States. All hospices were Christian, with the exception of the Jewish City of Hope Hospice in California (Small 1998). Hospice is now a term that describes both a place and a philosophy of care that can take place in a wide range of care settings. 'Hospice care' and 'palliative care' are terms that are commonly thought to be synonymous (Lawton 2000, 18); however, palliative care rather than hospice care is more widely used since the development of the medical specialism of palliative medicine, a development that is discussed later in this chapter.

Developments in the United Kingdom

In the United Kingdom the current model of hospice care is one that has developed from the work of Dame Cicely Saunders. In the 1960s Saunders and other medical professionals became disillusioned with the care of dying patients in hospitals. Saunders established St Christopher's Hospice in London. St Christopher's is a community 'inspired and informed by Christianity' (Small 1998, 170). The community was described by Saunders as 'the kind of family and home that can give the kind of welcome and hospitality of a good home' (Saunders 1965). The ideal of the hospice movement was to provide a form of extended family which sought to give patients a more personal form of care and which stressed the importance of including the family as well as the dying person within the remit of care (DuBois 1980).

St Christopher's quickly became a model for future developments, inspiring other groups of people across the UK to set up their own services (Lunt 1985, 753). While the hospice philosophy is rooted in a Christian tradition, Saunders was also influenced by the work of Victor Frankl (1985). Frankl developed Logotherapy, which focuses on the meaning of human existence and the human search for meaning. It is based on his own experiences in a Nazi concentration camp. Frankl puts forward a view that meaning can be found in life even when we are confronted with hopeless situations. 'When we are no longer able to change a situation—just think of an incurable disease such as inoperable cancer—we are challenged to change ourselves' (*op. cit.*, 135). Frankl argues that when there is no way out of suffering then we have a responsibility for the attitude in which we suffer. No one can tell another the meaning of his life, and what people need is the time and opportunity to find their own meaning. Frankl's ideas concerning an individual search for meaning have been highly influential, particularly on changing understandings of the concept of spirituality (Small 1998, 174).

Other influences

While the development of hospice care in the United Kingdom is rooted in a Christian tradition, there are other ways of understanding the end of life and responses to it that exist alongside a spiritual one. The study of death and dying also draws on work within psychology and psychiatry; Freud and Jung have been influential in addition to the existential philosophy of Frankl (Small 1998, 174).

A key figure in the area of death and dying, particularly in the United States, is Elisabeth Kübler-Ross and there are elements of the psychological, the spiritual and the existential in her work. Kübler-Ross was critical of the Cartesian mind/body split and promoted holistic care of dying people (*ibid.*, 175). Like Saunders in the UK, Kübler-Ross observed the isolation of dying patients and a lack of attention to their needs. She developed a stage theory of dying, based on work with over 200 dying patients, and observed that, in coming to terms with a terminal illness, many patients went through stages of denial, anger, bargaining, depression and acceptance (Kübler-Ross 1970).

The stage theory developed by Kübler-Ross was very influential in understanding the experiences and needs of dying people, especially for nurse training (Walter 1994, 72). Copp (1998) maintained that Kübler-Ross's theory gained acceptance largely because it filled a void in health care theory. Questions have been raised, however, about the adequacy and validity of this stage theory (Weisman 1974; Charmaz 1980; Kastenbaum 1985). A major criticism is that it is too mechanistic an approach as it fails to consider that while in practice most dying people experience all of these stages, they may not follow any order or they may not experience all of the stages. Dying people may also move in and out of these feelings at different times or they may experience several of them at the same time. Young and Cullen (1996) considered these stages in relation to patients in their study and felt that by and large they did not fit their experience. They argued that any conceptualisation also needs to take account of age, and that the degree of individualism is so great that any one conceptualisation cannot be applied to all (*op. cit.*, 16).

Changes and developments in palliative care

The setting up of hospices outside the NHS was intended by Saunders to demonstrate a quality of care that would eventually change standards within the NHS (Walter 1994, 169). Saunders has stated that hospices were developed outside the NHS 'in order to move back in' (Taylor 1983, cited in James and Field 1992). St Christopher's Hospice was opened in 1967, by which time it had already received a grant from the Ministry of Health for a home care service (although this was not established until 1969). An outpatient department was also initiated in 1969 (James and Field 1992, 1367). By 1976 Saunders wrote that 'the growth of what has become known as the "hospice movement" now shows about 20 homes for terminal care throughout the UK and a dozen Marie Curie homes' (Saunders 1976).

While it was Saunders's intention that improved care for dying people and their relatives should become part of the mainstream, the form and structures of these improvements have been shaped by a number of factors. Ideological changes in the welfare state under Thatcherism and reforms in the NHS since 1991 have brought palliative care services further into the NHS organisational framework (Small 1998, 18) and brought the language of audit, quality, cost effectiveness and so on into the hospice 'business'.

James and Field (1992) have examined the routinisation and bureaucratisation of the hospice movement in an English context and argued that some of the changes and reforms have come from within the hospice movement but that others, such as the establishment of palliative medicine as a speciality (by the Royal College of Physicians in 1987), have led to an increase in the medical imperative to intervene and this marks a move away from the earlier, more holistic, hospice model. The re-medicalisation of hospices is exemplified by the change in terminology from 'terminal care' to palliative medicine and the career-based developments of doctors specialising in 'palliative medicine'. James and Field argued that in some circumstances physical care dominates over social, psychological and spiritual care (1992, 1373). Furthermore, Bradshaw (1996b) suggested that the secularisation of the original ideals and the specialism of palliative care alter the original relationship of care and allow the techniques of various experts, medical and therapeutic, to predominate. Thus, 'death is no longer a truth to be confronted but a process to be managed' (1996b, 418).

A dual process of expansion and incorporation

James and Field have argued that the process of social change has meant that hospices affected, and were affected by, the structures of terminal care to which they were, and continue to be, a response (1992, 1373). This process of social change is reflected in a dual process of expansion and incorporation of palliative care within existing health care provision and beyond.

Hospice or palliative care is now present in almost every industrialised country in the world. The experience of establishing some of these services is recounted in a volume, edited by Saunders and Kastenbaum (1997), in which every continent (and 21 countries) is represented, demonstrating the global spread of palliative care in a relatively short period of time.

According to a study by Voltz *et al.* (1997), the number of hospice programmes in the US in 1997 was roughly 1700. In Germany the first hospice institution was opened in 1983 and at the time of the study there were 21 palliative care units and eleven in-patient hospices. In Japan the hospice idea was first introduced by Christian and Buddhist initiatives but has now been taken over by the national health system. The first in-patient palliative care unit was established in 1981. By 1995 the government had approved fourteen palliative care units and in-patient hospices.

In a recent comparative survey of the development of palliative care in seven European countries—UK, Sweden, Italy, Germany, Spain, Belgium and the Netherlands (Clark 2000)—differences were found in the initial time-frame of establishing these services. Initiatives took place between 1967 and 1991, with the elements of palliative care being established at various times. For example, Sweden established a home care service in 1977, home care was established in Italy in 1980, and Spain established an in-patient palliative care unit within a hospital in 1984. Clark noted that the extent to which palliative care is developing as a specialism also varies considerably, although this tends to reflect the degree of palliative care services or the relative affluence of specific countries (*op. cit.*, 442). Clark also noted that palliative care services in most European countries have only reached an initial stage of integration with the formal health care system.

While formal integration into health care systems is at an early stage in most European countries, the development of hospital-based palliative care services has been established in the UK since 1977; by 1996 approximately 160 hospitals had palliative care services (McQuillan *et al.* 1996). Palliative care services are now considered at different levels of ascending specialisation: level one is the palliative care approach in which the principles of palliative care can be applied by all health professionals; level two is general palliative care which, at an intermediate level, may be available from a range of health care professionals who have had some additional training and expertise in palliative care; and level three is specialist palliative care, i.e. services that are limited to the provision of palliative care—the original hospice model (NCH-SPCS 1996).

A current challenge for palliative care is the extension of the service to other, non-cancer, patients which has been advocated since 1980 (Wilkes 1980). Addington-Hall and Higginson (2001) have outlined the current arguments for inclusion of other patient groups. The physical, emotional and spiritual needs of dying patients and their families are not exclusive to cancer patients, and cancer patients cannot be considered to have a monopoly on suffering (Wasson and George 2001, 240). The aims of palliative care, such as holistic care, maintaining quality of life and dignity, family and carer support, are seen as equally applicable to non-cancer patients. The exclusion of non-cancer patients from palliative care services has raised issues of equity and has become indefensible on ethical grounds.

Underlying principles of palliative care

Lawton (2000) has argued that the modern hospice movement formed part of a broader cluster of social movements that shared a number of features. There is, according to Lawton, a distinct parallel between the hospice and the alternative health movement as both advocate that the patient should be seen as a 'whole person' (2000, 14). There are also parallels with the women's health movement, which challenged the technological focus of modern medicine, particularly in relation to childbirth; this has already been discussed in relation to the natural death movement as part of the attempt to medicalise death. The holistic view of the patient and the emphasis on death as a natural event have shaped and informed the principles of palliative care, which are open awareness and communication and the concept of 'total pain'.

Communication and open awareness

Both Saunders and Kübler-Ross formulated ways to understand the experiences and needs of dying people and how they could be addressed—through communication, listening and supporting both the patient and the family. Alongside the work of Saunders and Kübler-Ross, others such as Glaser and Strauss (1965) were influential in the debate on communication and awareness about dying in modern western societies. The Glaser and Strauss study—*Awareness of dying*—was based on research into the organisation of dying in San Francisco Bay area hospitals and concerned the way in which awareness about death was managed and communicated.

Glaser and Strauss identified four 'awareness contexts'—closed awareness, where staff kept patients ignorant of their impending death; suspicion awareness, where patients suspected that they were dying and tried to get staff and relatives to confirm this suspicion; mutual pretence, where all parties knew that the patient was dying but did not acknowledge this, pretending that 'everything was normal'; and open awareness, where all parties knew about and acknowledged that the patient was dying and were therefore able to talk about it.

Since the 1960s there has been a considerable shift from closed awareness to open awareness. This trend is particularly evident in the United States. For instance, a study published in 1961, 'What to tell cancer patients' (Oken 1961), showed that 88% of doctors would not normally tell cancer patients their diagnosis. Novak *et al.* (1979) replicated this study in the 1970s and found that 98% of respondents would usually tell their patients the prognosis.

There are several reasons why open awareness about death and dying became more common and why it is currently considered very important in palliative care. Improved health care, and in particular improvements in the treatment of cancer, makes a prognosis clearer; it also means that many people spend a longer time living with incurable illness. As a result, it can be more difficult to hide the truth about a terminal illness, or at least more difficult to manage non-disclosure (Walter 1994, 32). McNamara *et al.* (1994) contend that while formalised hospice objectives do not state disclosure norms regarding impending death, open communication concerning death seems to be the 'preferred interaction between patients and nurse and a path toward a "good death".

The practice of establishing open awareness about death and dying is most clearly seen in the United States, as the Novak *et al*. study shows. A change in the legislation enforcing the patient's right to informed consent has ensured that patients are informed about why treatment is needed, and consequently there can be open discussion about the illness and prognosis (Field and Copp 1999). Young and Cullen (1996, 112) have described the situation in the United Kingdom as one of transition. Drawing on other studies (for example Davey 1988, conference presentation cited in Young and Cullen), they described a situation of 'benevolent paternalism', where some doctors are willing to tell patients that they have suffered a heart attack or heart failure but are reluctant to disclose information about cancer. Some doctors assume that if patients do not ask they do not want to be told, 'especially so if patients were elderly, working class and poorly educated', adding weight to the view that the means of negotiating a 'good death' are not evenly distributed.

Conditional awareness

Walter (1994) has argued that a transfer of authority from the Church and from medicine to the individual has fuelled a revolution in attitudes to death and dying. A commitment to open awareness and communication is the norm in the USA, as discussed, a move driven by legislative change. In the UK there has been a similar though more gradual change (Field and Copp 1999). Seale *et al*. (1997) have stated that 'a preference for open awareness of dying is now well established in terminal care settings and amongst the general populations in the UK, USA and other Anglophone countries'. Young and Cullen (1996, 104) report on a study conducted by Dr L. Fallowfield at the Royal London Hospital in which researchers asked patients whether, prior to a consultation, they wished to have all the information, whether good or bad; information only if it were good; or whether they wanted to leave it up to the doctor. Ninety-five per cent of people wanted all the information, 3% wanted the information only if it was good news and 2% wanted the doctor to decide.

Field and Copp (1999) suggest that in spite of an ideological commitment to open awareness and a wish for full information, there seems to have been a progression from closed to open awareness and then partially back to 'conditional awareness'. This means that whilst there is now recognition that patients and family have a right to full information and may wish to have this, they may be unwilling to be continually reminded that they are dying even though they know this is the case (1999, 466). Hinton (1999), in a study of the progress of awareness and acceptance of dying in cancer patients and their relatives, also found an individual and fluctuating response to awareness of impending death, with awareness generally increasing as death approached, but some patients and one relative in the study also showed decreased awareness (1999, 25). Field and Copp (1999, 465) argue that the consequences and implications of this position may create emotional and professional tensions which doctors and nurses must manage in such a way as to facilitate informed patient choice.

Cultural differences

There are considerable cultural differences with regard to the appropriateness of open awareness about death and dying. Seale (1998) argues that the Anglo-American culture of individualism is at the heart of the growth of the patient-centred approach to relationships between health professionals and patients. However, in other cultures there is not necessarily the same individualism. In Japan, for instance, there is an expectation that doctors will make decisions on behalf of patients without sharing the thinking behind the decision, and family members often make decisions on behalf of another family member (1998, 111).

A study conducted in Italy (Surbone 1992) argues that this idea of patient autonomy is, in an Italian context, considered as patient and social isolation. In this context the protection of the patient by the family, considered negatively as collusion or denial in awareness contexts (Faulkner *et al.* 1994), is understood as protection and as shouldering the burden of knowledge for the patient (Seale 1998, 112).

In an Irish study, 'Telling the truth about cancer: views of elderly patients and their relatives' (*Irish Medical Journal*, 2000), of 120 patients, 83% of patients wanted to be told the truth and 55% of relatives wanted their next of kin informed; there was agreement between patients and relatives in 61% of cases. The usual reason given by relatives for not wanting the patient to know was that it would cause worry or depression. These findings would seem to indicate that Ireland is closer to the European model of truth-telling than to the North American one.

The concept of 'total pain'

The palliative care model is the holistic care of the patient and the family and encompasses four dimensions: emotional, physical, social and spiritual. It operates to a holistic model of pain incorporating the idea of 'total pain'—pain is present on the physical, emotional, social and spiritual levels (Baines 1990, 26). This concept was developed from the work of Saunders, who observed that once the physical symptoms and pain were managed and controlled, patients often revealed their emotional, psychological or spiritual concerns about death and dying. The concept of 'total pain' is also a development of the Gestaltian idea that a dying person's physical, emotional, social and spiritual concerns are inextricably entwined and each contributes to a 'total pain experience' (Lawton 2000, 13). It is understood, however, that physical pain often masks pain on other levels, or that emotional or social pain can exacerbate physical pain (Baines 1990, 28).

The incorporation of the psychological and spiritual concerns of individuals into the medical model can be seen not only as a way of offering better care but also as an extension of control (Arney and Bergen 1984). Palliative care sets out to provide total care of the dying person and his/her family but it has been argued that 'total care' may be 'total control'. In 'Total pain: disciplinary power and the body in the work of Cicely Saunders', Clark (1999) argued that total pain is a paradox. On the one hand it seems to humanise physical suffering and acknowledges that pain has to be understood as something including, but greater than, physical matters of sensation. Freeing patients from physical pain can provide access to their other problems, mental, spiritual and social. On the other hand, as Clark suggests, there is also something imperialistic about the notion of 'total pain', where an initial focus on the physical sensation of pain leads to a wider and deeper search for signs of trouble, in the social network, in the psyche, even in the soul itself.

This is an inherent paradox in the critique of medicalisation—if medicine takes the social aspects of health and illness into account it is accused of medical imperialism; if it does not it is accused of medical reductionism (Nettleton 1995, 157). This type of critique is influenced by the work of Foucault and his conceptualisation of the 'clinical gaze' (Foucault 1976), in which he argues that the patient is constructed under the 'clinical gaze' of the physician and reduced to the pathologies displayed. Foucault's later (1982) development of 'pastoral power' offers another way to consider developments toward holism in modern medicine. Pastoral power is a form of surveillance that directs its gaze inward toward people as individual subjects rather than as objects, and which, according to Foucault, implies knowledge of the consciousness and an ability to direct it. The conjoining of these two words suggests that the traditional pastoral concerns of the clergy have become generalised and redirected toward health and well-being (McGowen 1994). As McGowen explains, pastoral power claims the loyalty of the subject precisely because 'it promises to foster and respect the liberated individual whom it pretends to have discovered' (1994, 100).

Pastoral power may be a dynamic present in the concept of total pain, a dynamic that leads to an assumption that all dying people have multi-dimensional concerns that need to be addressed, and an obligation may be placed on the dying person to embrace death as a 'final stage of growth'. Lofland (1978) has described this perspective as the 'happy death movement'. A component of this ideal is that death offers the opportunity for last-minute perfection, and for the dying person to suppress the expression of their spiritual pain is 'to sacrifice the opportunities for growth which death provides' (1978, 99).

Multi-disciplinary team working

In order to address the multi-dimensional aspects of pain, palliative care draws on the expertise of different professionals. Abu-Saad states that the goal of multi-disciplinary palliative care is the provision of excellent care, taking into consideration the complexity of care provided, the utilisation of the appropriate skills provided by the team members and minimisation of fragmentation of care (2001, 21). According to Abu-Saad, the dynamic of multi-disciplinary team working is one of mutuality, respect and interdependence. Coyle (1997, cited in Abu-Saad 2001) has listed a number of barriers to team working in palliative care, such as the culture of the organisation, the hierarchical authority of the physician in relation to the nurse, issues regarding 'ownership' of the patient, and the question of expertise with regard to profession, service and team. Confusion about the different roles and boundaries between the roles of team members can also cause difficulties (Abu-Saad 2001, 21).

Professional roles of team members

Multi-disciplinary teams consist of doctors, nurses, social workers and chaplains, although the range and numbers of professional staff differ from service to service and are dependent on available resources. Multi-disciplinary teams also have close involvement with the families of dying patients (Baines 1990, 33).

The health professionals with whom patients and families have most contact are nurses, and nurses play a key role in the team (Abu-Saad 2001). The close and continuing contact with the patient gives the nurse an opportunity to observe the patient in pain, observations which are crucial for pain diagnosis and treatment (Baines 1990, 34).

The role of the nurse in the palliative care team is more blurred than that of the other team members. This is partly due to the skills nurses have in terms of symptom control and psychosocial care, but also because of the intuitive learned experience of nursing dying people and caring for families in general (Dunlop and Hockley 1998).

Physicians on the team deal, in general, with complex symptom control as well as issues relating to the patients' and families' understanding of the diagnosis and prognosis. It is also the responsibility of physicians to clarify difficulties with end-of-life decision-making with the team, patients and relatives, and to reflect and debate, with other team members, on current medical management of patients who are terminally ill (Abu-Saad 2001, 22).

The social worker assesses and advises on the psychological, emotional and social problems of patients and their families. The assessment of family attitudes and resources forms an integral part of the treatment plan for patients, and the social worker uses individual or group work techniques in the assessment process (*ibid.*, 23).

The chaplain appears to have a peripheral role in the palliative care team, although Abu-Saad (2001) states that there are a number of important roles for the chaplain—sorting out religious or spiritual issues, acting as a patient advocate by taking the patient's and family's perspective, and guidance on ethical decisions and problems. Counselling patients and providing bereavement follow-up services are also seen as core activities for the chaplain in the clinical environment (*ibid.*, 23). A discussion of the role of chaplains in the context of spiritual care is presented in the section on spirituality and spiritual care.

A 'good death' in palliative care

Bradbury's study (1999) has considered contemporary ideas of a 'good death' for a variety of people and settings connected with death and dying. A 'good death' within palliative care provides a specific context for considering a 'good death', a context that has been shaped by the development of palliative care within cancer care. With many more people living longer with terminal illness, palliative care is focused on enabling people to live their final years and months more fully and consciously.

Kellehear (2001) suggested a number of aspects that are important for a 'good death'— adjusting to the different cycles of illness and treatment, the legal, financial and religious preparations for death, disengagement from work and the bidding of farewells. In a review of the literature Mak and Clinton (1999) suggest that a 'good death' involves a complex set of relations and preparations that are not separate acts but a series of social events (McNamara *et al*. 1995).

Mak and Clinton establish that comfort and relief from pain and suffering are among the most commonly cited elements of a 'good death' (Nimocks *et al.* 1987; Weisman 1988; WHO 1990, amongst others). The emphasis on freedom from pain accounts to some degree, according to Mak and Clinton, for a confusion between a 'good death' and euthanasia. Palliative care emphasises that the sufferings of the patient should be reduced and that troublesome and debilitating symptoms should be controlled to enable a 'good death' (Mak and Clinton 1999, 100). The World Health Organisation also states that freedom from pain is an essential element of a 'good death' in order to leave the patient physically and mentally 'capable of reaching whatever goals he or she may want to achieve before death' (WHO 1990).

Additional aspects of a 'good death' include completion—death can be seen as essentially 'good' when it occurs 'on time', when a person has completed their span of life or has a sense of readiness related to their style of life and to their aspirations and goals in life (Hinton 1967; Shneidman 1973). Acceptance and autonomy are further elements of a good death identified by Mak and Clinton (1999), although achieving acceptance can be a gradual process. This process begins when the patient becomes aware of impending death, but as death becomes closer people may need help in giving meaning to their lives (from Weisman 1972 and Nimocks *et al*. 1987). A 'good death' in this sense, according to Mak and Clinton, is one in which patients accept they are at the end of their lives but believe that their lives had meaning (Mak and Clinton 1999, 102).

Additional aspects of a 'good death' are the public preparations for death, saying farewell to the family and staff (Kellehear 1990; Smith and Maher 1993). It is also important to complete 'unfinished business'—by making personal and social preparations including resolving residual conflicts and satisfying remaining wishes (Weisman 1972). These elements of a 'good death' are supported by a study by Steinhauser *et al*. (2000) which identified six themes that characterised a 'good death': pain and symptom management, clear decision-making, preparation for death, completion, contributing to others, and affirmation of the whole person. Steinhauser *et al.* also noted distinct differences between groups (patients, family members, physicians, nurses, social workers, chaplains and volunteers), which were shaped by social and professional roles (2000, 829).

A 'good death' for whom?

Dekkers *et al.* suggest that the characteristics of a 'good death' might not be all about the person dying (2002, 113) and advocate that the views of the family and health care personnel should also be included, although these may be in conflict with what is good for the dying person. This difference in perspective may be reflected in the views of the dying and the caregivers. For caregivers, the focus of attention can be on how 'comfortable' the passage of illness and death is and how satisfactory the carers feel their care has been for the dying person (Kellehear 2001, 210).

A comparative study of the views of hospice staff and patients on perceptions of a 'good death' showed a divergence between patients and staff (Payne and Langley-Evans 1996) in addition to common features shared by patients, families and professionals. Patients were more concerned with dying quietly, preferably during sleep, or even dying suddenly, whereas staff were more concerned with a lack of physical pain, presence of the family and that the patient should show no anxiety.

Payne and Langley-Evans suggest that one reason for the disparity may be a different focus—emphasis on symptom control is part of the medical model and the perspective of staff may function to maintain the organisational stability of hospice work, and in doing so may constrain patterns of dying.

Spirituality and spiritual care

Spiritual care is one dimension of the multi-dimensional approach of palliative care, as already discussed. A definition of spirituality is difficult to establish. There have been continuous debates, which can be documented in the palliative care literature over the last eighteen years (Baird 1985; Roy 1987; Saunders 1988; Bown and Williams 1993; Babler 1997; Dom 1999; Hopper 2000, amongst others), about the differences between spirituality and religion and about what constitutes spirituality.

This discussion seems, at times, to circle endlessly around definitions of spirituality without any satisfactory resolution. In the context of palliative care it is a critical area for definition as it not only affects the dying person but also has organisational implications. Who can provide spiritual care cannot be ascertained until a clear definition of what it is has been reached.

The problem of definition

Roy (1987) suggests that the term 'spiritual' seems reserved to cover vaguely what is left over after physicians, pain control experts, nurses, psychologists, counsellors and therapists have given the best they have to offer the dying. In spite of all that has been discussed concerning spiritual care in the intervening years definition remains a problem, although a theoretical model proposed by Kellehear (2000b) (discussed below) brings some clarity. One approach has been to understand it as a search for meaning (Speck 1998). This interpretation builds on the work of Victor Frankl, and has become generally accepted. This definition can be helpful; people who hold unorthodox or no religious beliefs can still be seen to have needs beyond the physical, emotional and social aspects of care. It removes the spiritual care of the dying from a strictly religious realm and enables spiritual care to be provided by anyone for anyone (Walter 1997, 25), in theory at least. If spirituality is defined as an individual search for meaning, however, then meaning, if it is uncovered, is individualistic. This can lead to difficulties as to what is needed and who can provide it.

Speck (1998) outlines some useful definitions of the spirituality, religious and philosophical dimensions as follows. Spirituality is considered a search for existential meaning within a life experience, with reference to a power other than the self, which may or may not be called God. Religious is a particular system of faith and worship expressive of an underlying spirituality and interpretative of the named religious understanding of God. When the search for meaning excludes any reference to a power other than the individual it can be considered as philosophical. Life events and the destiny of the individual are seen as manifestations of the individual's own personality as expressed individually or corporately. This does not mean that they are seen as totally separated from each other: for instance, all those belonging to a subset 'religious' would also belong to a subset 'spiritual', but those who are spiritual would not necessarily express that in a religious way. Some of those within the philosophy set will also be spiritual and some will not.

A theoretical model

Speck's definitions can also be usefully applied to the theoretical model that Kellehear proposes, which is based on the idea that human beings have a desire to transcend hardship and suffering (2000b, 150). Stated in this way, this model builds on the understanding of spirituality as an individual search for meaning. Kellehear suggests, however, that people search for meaning in different situations, contexts and beliefs, and these can also overlap. In fact Kellehear suggests that there can be considerable interaction between them, depending on the particular social and cultural background of the person. His proposed model features three basic aspects. The first consists of situational needs, which involve making sense of life—seen by many as a central task of spirituality. This is particularly pertinent and crucial to the task of 'making the most' of living with dying. These attitudes and values assist in promoting a personal sense of the quality of life and also touch on such areas as hope, companionship and 'being there', all aspects of the current debates on spirituality.

The second aspect comprises moral and biographical needs that concern changes in a person's situation and which may in turn give rise to other needs that may not be directly addressed by religious or theological discourses but may be related to religion. There have been a limited number of studies looking at the role of religion and coping in chronic illness. Those that have been conducted suggest that religion is a common coping mechanism that may have positive effects in relation to adjustment (Dein 1997, 295). Kellehear argues that much of the content and direction of these needs and questions can be found in parallel concerns in traditional religious discourses. In broad cultural terms, the language and structure of some of these needs frequently reflect the language and structure of the same questions in religious discourse (*op. cit.*, 151).

The final aspect of Kellehear's model concerns religious needs that may arise out of autobiographical reflections (*op. cit.*, 152). The person may have existing religious beliefs that now need to be interrogated on the basis of the new experience of dying or they may occur as a recent interest in questions of a religious nature. As Kellehear states, although there are current debates about secularisation in modern societies, religious questions are common among people, dying or not, and there may be a need to resolve unresolved religious questions and issues.

Attributes of spiritual care

Without a clear definition of spirituality it is difficult to ascertain what the attributes of spiritual care should be. Early writing by Saunders suggests that spiritual care is not so much a set of tasks as simply 'being there' (1965). Saunders draws on her own Christian faith and uses the example of Jesus in the Garden of Gethsemane, who asked his companions to 'watch with me'. Saunders considers the word 'watch' to be critical and suggests that it means a lot that cannot be understood; what it does not mean, she argues, is that it is necessary to 'understand what is happening' or 'explain' or 'take away' (*op. cit.*, 2). The approach promoted by Saunders includes helping patients to be free of pain and distress but also means being silent, listening and 'being there'. Saunders (1988) suggests that it is often the practical tasks—caring for the physical needs, time taken to clarify a symptom and the quiet acceptance of a family's demands—that reach the 'most hidden places' (*op. cit.*, 5).

Stanworth (1997) also explores attributes of spiritual care, suggesting that much of what is expressed in spirituality is done through symbolic gestures and metaphors, and argues that the 'vocabulary of the spirit belongs to a language of depth and meaning unfolds in the context of relationship', rather than being available for detached analysis (*op. cit.*, 20). Czechmeister has also argued that the feelings experienced by patients are often 'beyond words' (1994, 1232). Given the literal translation of metaphor (from the Greek) as 'going beyond', metaphorical language is an effective way to understand the phenomenological world of the patient and the experience of illness (*ibid.*, 1232).

Stanworth emphasises the relationship aspect of spiritual care, advocating the need 'to see with the eye of the heart' (1997, 22). Arguing that this relationship is often expressed though symbolic language and metaphor, Stanworth draws on examples of poetic language which she suggests triumphs through its relationship with life—one of interaction rather than observation and management.

Roy also subscribes to this connection with poetry and poetic language, stating that 'poets capture and perpetuate in word and rhythm those seemingly simple and everyday experiences that make real and tie together a lifetime's worth of meaning' (1999, 4). The ability to hear patients, Stanworth argues, is dependent upon being willing and prepared to risk uncertainty and 'to travel with them to places where there is no expert vocabulary to protect us' (1997, 22).

Stanworth's (1997) focus on relationship places demands on professionals working in palliative care. Saunders (1988), however, states that those caring for the dying are not the only givers. Carers, according to Saunders, receive as much as they give, but there is a need to embark on their own search for meaning and spiritual journey because unless they do so they will be unable to help patients (*op. cit.*, 4).

Cornette (1997) in a large-scale study in Belgium focused on the spiritual needs of caregivers. The study established an assumption that patients, their partners and volunteers suffered the most spiritual distress, followed by those involved in pastoral care. Physicians were considered to have the lowest level of spiritual distress. The study found, however, that physicians rated their own spiritual distress as high. Cornette argued that 'stubborn preconceptions' about professional roles appear to prevent caregivers from offering good spiritual care to each other and that 'in the face of death professional masks and uniforms tend to slip and questions about the meaning of life and death are stealing upon all disciplines of caregivers' (*op. cit.*, 11). Respondents to the study considered the ability to discern one's own spiritual needs and to develop self-awareness to be important criteria for spiritual care of patients. Cornette argued that spiritual care involves watching, listening and accepting patients just as they are, and these aspects of spiritual care apply equally to professional colleagues and to caring for oneself (*op. cit.*, 13).

Delivering spiritual care

Cobb stated that there is a dichotomy between the general ideals of palliative care and the reality of practice, which is both an internal debate of the specialism and a debate in the wider cultural and sociological contexts (2001, 125). Cobb argued that spiritual care moves beyond the conventional approach dependent on expertise and into an encounter between two vulnerable human beings alert to the creative possibilities of transcendence (*op. cit.*, 126).

Kellehear's (2000b) model suggest, however, that religious needs are an important part of spiritual care, and that religious needs and issues are still pertinent for the spiritual care of the dying. This raises the question of who can provide this care. Pastoral care has traditionally been provided by hospital and hospice chaplains. This is still the case, although with increasing secularisation the position of the chaplain may be eroded. The palliative model of care demands that all members of the multi-disciplinary team be alert to all aspects of the patient's needs.

Nurses are well placed to provide the kind of spiritual care that is promoted by Saunders—that of listening and 'being there'. The debate that can be documented in the UK and palliative care nursing literature demonstrates that many nurses may feel inadequate and unsure of their abilities, and can also feel that this type of care is outside the remit of nursing (Burnard 1987; Sodestrom and Martinson 1987; Herth 1990; Mak 1992; Ross 1997, amongst others). McSherry (2001, 113), however, has argued that nurses can distinguish between a spiritual need that has its origins within a religious framework and those that are more existential in nature. Cobb asserts that, in spite of a change in nursing towards a liberal humanism at the expense of its theological and pastoral base in the 1970s (Bradshaw 1996b), spiritual care has been rediscovered and reinterpreted as another aspect of the knowledge and role of the nurse (Cobb 2001, 77).

The role of the chaplain

The multi-disciplinary nature of palliative care has developed and in some ways expanded but also eroded the role of the chaplain. Ainsworth-Smith (1998) outlined the changes in this role and sees the function of the chaplain as a much wider one, serving organisational needs as much as those of individuals. He considers that the work of the chaplain is focused in three areas—the patients and their relatives, the hospital staff and trainees, and the needs of the organisation. The needs of the patients and their families are seen as addressing religious and personal questions that arise from people being in a 'new unmapped place', and this may cause difficulties for staff and raise further questions of their own. On an organisational level, Ainsworth-Smith advocates that chaplains develop a 'bi-lingualism', that is, not only the language of a religious tradition but also discourses from psychology and sociology in order to have a wider view of organisational stress.

A view of the role of the chaplain in wider health care contexts is offered by Carr (2001), who considers the role as manager, arbiter, facilitator and interpreter. Carr suggests that the chaplain needs to manage the worship or liturgical aspects of the health care community, including patients and staff, who have become a form of 'temporary parish'. This identifies the basic religious aspect of the chaplain's role, through which the chaplain can explore issues of thanksgiving and despair that often surface in health care settings but especially so in hospices (*op. cit.*, 29). Carr suggests that a chaplain, in lieu of multi-faith ministries, can act as an arbiter for all religious practice. Although Carr acknowledges that this may be a controversial stance, the reality of a lack of people engaged in ministry and financial restrictions within health care has led in practice to chaplains adopting the role of arbiter. The chaplain also acts as facilitator, according to Carr, largely because of the loose relationship of chaplaincy with health care organisational structures—the chaplain often occupies any place structurally within health care settings. Carr uses an interesting example of chaplaincy within the Royal Navy, where the chaplain is regarded as holding the rank of the person to whom he is speaking (*op. cit.*, 30). Linked to this loose organisational relationship, Carr argues that the role of chaplaincy is also one of interpreter. Because of the ambiguous position of the chaplain (between centre and margin, between religion and spirituality, between institutional role and the person) the chaplain may be in a privileged position to be used as an interpreter for the institution for what may be happening to people (*op. cit.*, 30). Carr argues that there is a further role for the chaplain in contributing to the spiritual and ethical issues that arise in health care, both personal and institutional. In this sense chaplains are caretakers of the personal and institutional values.

Inequitable representation

Orchard (2001) has surveyed chaplaincy in London hospitals to establish which religious denominations are represented—a question, she suggests, not so much of 'being there' as of 'who is not there'. Acknowledging that London is the most ethnically diverse of all UK cities (Storkey 1993, cited in Orchard 2001) and that ethnicity is a poor indicator of religious affiliation, Orchard maintains that the spiritually cosmopolitan nature of the capital is evidenced by the listings of certified places of worship affiliated to different religious groups. The multi-faith directory (Weller 1997, cited in Orchard 2001) lists 395 Muslim, 213 Hindu, 183 Jewish and 42 Sikh organisations and worship centres in the Greater London area. In contrast to this, Orchard's analysis of funded chaplaincy sessions in London NHS Trust hospitals revealed that funded chaplaincy sessions to faiths other than Christian are under 6%, with no funded sessions allocated to six of Britain's nine major faith groups (Orchard 2001, 149). Orchard also reveals that for non-funded positions such as volunteers and visiting ministers the presence of minority faiths is sparse.

Orchard dismisses the financial constraints as justifiable reasons for this lack of representation as, according to Orchard, even when funding is available there are other obstacles. These obstacles are the tendency of Christian chaplains, particularly Anglicans, to assume the role of spiritual broker on behalf of all faiths, in addition to representing their own. This impacts on the formal mechanism for including others on the team, diminishes awareness of the need for religious leaders from other faiths, and carries a risk of being patronising and exclusive (*op. cit.*, 152). The domination of an exclusively Christian view of spirituality is not confined to the provision of chaplaincy services, as Narayanasamy (1999) has established. A review of the nursing literature revealed that when spirituality is discussed in nursing it is almost exclusively treated from a Christian theological perspective, suggesting that the inequitable representation is not in terms of a physical presence but translates across and through professional discourses.

An additional obstacle is one of administrative and managerial ease. It is considered easier from a management perspective—recruitment and lines of accountability are clear—to maintain Christian chaplains as brokers or arbiters, as Carr (2001) identifies the role.

The under-representation of minority faiths in chaplaincy is also indicated in a survey of hospitals in England and Wales by Wright (2001), who argued that the role of chaplain is almost exclusively Christian and dominated by the Church of England. Orchard argues that this structural inequity results in an absence of choice for many patients and families and for many it is a case of making the best of what is on offer, which may actually increase existing difficulties (2001, 157). Addressing the under-representations of minority faiths in chaplaincy in health care is, according to Orchard, essential if patients and families are to be cared for in ways 'that genuinely meet their needs on their own terms' (*op. cit.*, 158).

Summary

The concept of a 'good death' is almost universal and is linked to control over the biological event. Historically this was pursued through religious belief. In the contemporary western world, with the declining role of Christianity, science and technology have largely replaced faith as a means of making sense of mortality.

Contemporary representations of a 'good death' reveal a number of categories of a 'good death', all of which are open to individual and professional negotiation. Representations of a 'good death' can be considered as culturally prescribed ways to demarcate the social order.

Palliative care involves the total care of dying patients. The goal is the best possible quality of life for patients and their families. Control of pain and symptoms and of psychological, social and spiritual problems is paramount. Palliative care has developed from the work of Cicely Saunders, and is now incorporated into mainstream health services. A current challenge is the extension of these services to non-cancer patients.

A key concept of palliative care is 'total pain', which considers pain on physical, emotional, psychological and spiritual levels. Multi-disciplinary team working is the mechanism by which multi-dimensional pain can be observed and addressed. This concept has been criticised by some as imperialistic as it may exercise increased control over patients.

Open awareness and communication is a further key concept within palliative care. Glaser and Strauss's theory on awareness of death and dying has been influential, in addition to legislative changes in the United States, although there are cultural differences about the appropriateness of these aspects. Theories of death and dying have also been influenced by Kübler-Ross; however, her stage theory has also been criticised as being too mechanistic and as failing to take account of individual responses to death and dying.

A 'good death' in palliative care has been shaped by the focus of palliative care within cancer care. Freedom from pain and distressing symptoms is a crucial element in order to facilitate other related aspects such as preparation, acceptance and completion of personal and social tasks. There may be a divergence of views between patients, families and professional staff concerning definitions of a 'good death'.

Spiritual care is a dimension of palliative care that has been subjected to debates on definitions of spirituality and who can provide spiritual care. Spirituality may be an individual search for existential meaning with reference to a power other than the self, which may or may not be called God, and which may or may not include religious need or expression. A theoretical model (Kellehear 2000b) suggests that people search for meaning in different situations, contexts and beliefs, and these can also overlap and interact, depending on the particular social and cultural background of the person. 'Being there' and listening are attributes of spiritual care. Some commentators suggest that metaphorical or symbolic language and gestures can reveal spiritual distress in ways that everyday vocabulary may not.

Nurses are also in a position of closeness and intimacy with patients. Some nurses feel inadequate and ill-equipped to deal with spiritual distress, while others feel that this is a part of the nursing role that has been rediscovered. Spiritual care, however, is commonly seen as the domain of chaplaincy. The role of the chaplain is evolving to incorporate religious and spiritual care for patients, staff and the organisation. Under-representation of chaplains from minority faiths results in limited choice for patients and families and limited definitions of spiritual care.

CHAPTER 2
The Irish dimension

Introduction

Studies concerning definitions of a 'good death' and spiritual care have usually taken place within societies that have a different historicity and culture to Ireland. Much of this research has taken place within the UK. Ireland and the UK are not only geographically close but share a common language and an interwoven history. While the UK has been a highly industrialised and multi-ethnic society for a considerable time, Ireland has been, until very recently, a relatively poor country, with little or no indigenous industry and with large-scale emigration. Since the mid-1990s, however, the economic climate has changed, with immigration rather than emigration more common, and a multi-cultural society is beginning to emerge. These social changes have occurred rapidly over a very short period.

The previous chapter has considered a 'good death' as a way in which to 'make the end, the parting from human beings, when it comes, as easy and as pleasant as possible, for others as well as ourselves' (Elias 1985). A 'good death' within palliative care and the spiritual care dimension of that model of care were reviewed in order to assess to what extent they affect the manner of parting. This parting, however, is also shaped by cultural values, beliefs and practices.

This chapter will look at the aspects of Irish culture that may shape this parting; for example, spirituality and the problems of definition that have been discussed in the previous chapter may be conceptualised in Ireland as a 'Celtic spirituality'. The cultural rituals and beliefs around death and dying in Ireland suggest that there may be a distinct cosmology present. In this context, the central role of the Catholic Church in Irish society and in the development of the Irish health service and the current structures of palliative care in Ireland are considered.

A central position: the Catholic Church in Ireland

Any studies of cultural influences that have shaped Irish society have to begin with the Catholic Church in Ireland, which has had a long and interwoven history with the political development of the country. From the nineteenth century until the 1970s the Catholic Church played a critical role in developing and shaping the social institutions of the state and in so doing exerted a major influence on the lives of Irish people that is still in evidence.

In nineteenth-century Ireland the major institutions of the state were organised by the British administration. Social institutions such as schools and hospitals reflected a religious and cultural ethos that was considered by the Catholic Church to be at variance with the religious, cultural and moral values of the majority of the population. This led the Catholic Church to develop its own schools, universities and hospitals. At the same time lay organisations such as the Society of Saint Vincent de Paul and the Knights of Columbanus were established; these organisations concerned themselves with the moral and social welfare of Catholic citizens. The Knights of Columbanus were first established secretly to promote Catholic social principles and Catholic individuals in public and private organisations in which they were working (Bolster 1979). Lay groups and organisations have played a significant role in maintaining the position and influence of the Catholic Church in Ireland. Inglis (1998, 53) has stated that since Vatican II and the decline in vocations these lay organisations have played an even greater role. In 1983 there were 26 different Catholic lay organisations affiliated to the hierarchy's Lay Commission, with a total membership of over 300,000.

Inglis has argued that the powerful position of the Catholic Church in Ireland is unusual and is not reflected in other predominantly Catholic countries such as Italy or Spain. The development of Catholic social institutions, such as schools and hospitals, afforded the opportunity for a Catholic social élite to emerge. These institutions and organisations provided positions of power for Catholics who would not have considered becoming, nor would indeed have been allowed to become, involved in the institutions of the state prior to the formation of the Irish Free State in 1922. In addition, control of these key social institutions enabled the Church to exert considerable influence over almost every aspect of life in Ireland.

Spheres of control and influence

The control of education has meant that almost all Irish Catholics have been educated by the Catholic Church, and while the instruction may not have been given by a nun or priest it was generally given by a schoolteacher appointed and supervised by a member of a religious order or the clergy (Inglis 1998, 58). Until 1971 it was also considered a mortal sin for Catholics not to send their children to Catholic schools. The insistence on denominational education, in both the north and the south of Ireland, is one of the main reasons, Inglis argues, for the persistence of different cultural practices between Catholics and Protestants.

The role of Catholic religious orders in the development and organisation of health care services in Ireland since the late nineteenth century has been considerable (Breen *et al.* 1990; Inglis 1998). The Catholic Church had enormous influence in health care. The ownership and control of hospitals and the representation of Catholic religious personnel on the boards of public hospitals has meant that the Church has been able to exert considerable influence on the way medicine is practised, on training and teaching, on the appointment of staff and over hospital ethics (Inglis 1998, 226). This influence is now somewhat diminished, however; currently 26 of the 63 hospitals in the state are Catholic voluntary hospitals. Voluntary hospitals under Protestant management also existed in Ireland, the last of which, the Adelaide Hospital in Dublin, merged with two hospitals, one of which was a Catholic hospital, in 1996 in a new major hospital development in the south-west of the city.

A gradual decline

The power and influence of the Catholic Church in Ireland began to decline from the 1970s. Central to this decline is the fall in vocations; over a thirty-year period 1966–1996 there has been a fall of 92% (Inglis 1998, 212). For the ten-year period 1990–1999 the number of new entrants of religious sisters, brothers and clerics was 867 but the numbers departing the religious life were 981. The age profile of people in a professed religious life in Ireland also shows a large ageing population; only 11% are aged 50 or under (Breen 2001). Although there is a marked decline in vocations, Ireland still has a higher proportion of religious per head of population than any other European country. For example, in Ireland 0.38% of the population are engaged in a professed religious life, compared to 0.019% in the UK/Wales and 0.205% in Italy (Maxwell 2001).

The decline in religious vocations in Ireland is a major factor in the loss of influence. Inglis has argued that in the heyday of the Catholic Church in Ireland there was a 'priest, nun or brother in every corner of Irish society' (1998, 211), providing a form of surveillance very much in keeping with Foucault's (1976) conceptualisation. Priests, nuns and brothers presided over hospitals, orphanages, homes, hostels, hospices, reform schools and Irish homes. According to Inglis, like all good authority figures their supervision and control continued even in their absence, and 'the supervisory eye of the Church was internalised in the hearts and minds of Irish Catholics' (1998, 211).

The power and influence of the Catholic Church in key areas such as politics and health care has diminished although it has not disappeared. For instance, as recently as 1997 a vasectomy clinic in a public hospital in County Donegal was closed owing to objections from Catholic groups. Following a vote of the board of the Regional Health Board it was reopened. The Catholic Church has also lost considerable ground as the moral authority for the majority of the population, with voters going against the teachings of the Church on two main issues: abortion and divorce. Following two referenda (1983 and 1992) on abortion, the electorate voted (in 1992) in favour of the right to travel to another country to have an abortion and the right to information about abortion services outside Ireland (Smyth 1992). Divorce was introduced in 1995 following a referendum that year; the result was very close, with 50.3% voting in favour and 49.7% voting against.

Part of the reason for the erosion of the Catholic Church as a moral authority has been the revelations, since the mid-1990s, concerning sexual abuse and sexual scandals. Inglis (1998, 216) has pointed out that in 1987 there were no stories in the media concerning the personal sexual behaviour of priests and religious. In contrast, by 1996 stories of child sex abuse by priests and religious had become commonplace. By 1996 there was also an ongoing debate about the position and role of the Catholic Church in Irish society and the way it handled its own affairs. According to Inglis, 'suddenly the Church had lost its sacredness and became another interest group in civil society which is open to the same inspection as any other' (*op. cit.*, 217).

While the Catholic Church may now be 'another interest group' it still has considerable influence in the sphere of education, with few changes in the management structures of primary and secondary schools in Ireland. There have been struggles with the state over the establishment of the multi-denominational primary schools and the creation of non-denominational community colleges. Much of the educational infrastructure by way of land and buildings is owned by the Catholic Church, as is also the case for other religions, such as the Church of Ireland. However, the degree of influence over the curriculum has decreased, and the decline in numbers of religious sisters, brothers and priests has made it difficult to maintain a religious influence within schools.

Protestant Catholics

The decline in religious vocations would suggest that Ireland is becoming more secular. However, the results of the 1990 European Values Survey (Hornsby-Smith and Whelan 1994) revealed that Irish people had a weekly church attendance rate which was twice the European average (*op. cit.*, 21). In spite of low Mass attendance rates in other European countries, the survey also revealed that substantial proportions of Catholics in all countries derive comfort and strength from their religion. The figure in Ireland is highest at 85%, compared with Great Britain at 73% and Germany at 46% (*ibid.*, 39).

Hornsby-Smith and Whelan have argued that a new type of Catholic is emerging in Ireland. This new Catholic displays an informed appreciation of the value of the supernatural and sacramental life of the Church, including an increasing tendency to think in terms of a spirit or life force rather than a personal God. Between 1981 and 1990 there was an increase from 15% to 24% of people believing in the idea of God as 'some sort of spirit or life force' as opposed to the idea of God as a personal figure, a shift which occurred over all age groups and not just among a younger age group as might be expected (*op. cit.*, 35).

In addition, this new type of Catholic questions the Church's authority to speak on matters of personal morality or on government policy (*op. cit.*, 35). Inglis (1998, 203–8) argues that Irish Catholics are becoming more Protestant; that is, they are devising their own spiritual and moral path to salvation and no longer rely on the moral or religious authority of the Catholic Church.

Celtic spirituality

The shift toward the idea of God as a life force rather than a personal God is interesting as it may well fit closely with a type of spirituality that is considered unique to Ireland and other Celtic countries—'Celtic spirituality'. There is some theological basis for asserting a difference between the early Irish Church and the Church of Rome—the early Irish Church emphasised the presence and understanding of God in and through the rhythms of the seasons. This was a different, though not contrary, theological emphasis to the teachings of the Roman Church. O'Loughlin (2000, 16) has argued that any group of Christians who share a common culture and similar attitudes to the larger world beyond themselves will develop a distinctive local flavour to their Christianity. The early Irish Church incorporated to some extent the beliefs and practices of the indigenous population.

In the nineteenth century the Catholic Church struggled to establish Roman orthodoxy. Inglis argues that the Catholic Church, in attempting to control and dominate, systematically eliminated or assimilated religious languages, beliefs, practice and morals that were opposed to its position. In some cases this involved trying to eradicate pagan beliefs and unacceptable practices, for example the outlawing of wakes and lamenting the dead (O'Suilleabháin 1967, 139–41), which began as early as 1614 at the Synod of Armagh. Strong condemnation of wake practices, particularly the 'singing of lewd songs and the playing of obscene games' (*ibid.*, 146), continued from the seventeenth century to the early twentieth century, when the Synod of Maynooth in 1927 forbade absolutely 'the holding of unchristian and unseemly wakes' (*ibid.*, 154).

O'Suilleabháin comments that the enforcing of the episcopal decrees fell mainly on the shoulders of parish priests and their curates, and people were slow to discontinue traditional practices; he notes that clerical action was taken only when the games and other aspects of local wakes were possible occasions for scandal and these activities were, in practice, allowed to die out naturally (*op. cit.*, 157).

Inglis argues that any ethnographic study of religious life in Ireland would still find evidence of earlier beliefs (1998, 206). Taylor (1995) states that 'each time a new religious form takes shape it does so with pre-existing materials—language, objects, places and notions'. These beliefs, according to Taylor, are embodied in the landscape, the home and the language and are a cultural residue which does not go away either in the society or the individual.

The language of 'Celtic spirituality' places a heavy emphasis on nature, sacred places and healing. An example of one such publication is *Anam Cara: spiritual wisdom from the Celtic world* (O'Donoghue 1999). The publisher's remarks on the cover of the book state that:

> *'when St Patrick came to Ireland, he encountered the Celtic people and a flourishing spiritual tradition that had already existed for thousands of years .... the ancient Celtic reverence for the spirit in all things survives today, a vibrant legacy of mystical wisdom that is unique in the Western World*'.

This is the language of marketing and publicity and has little historical accuracy.

It is arguable whether a unified Celtic people ever existed. While there is an image of the Celts as a people who are mystical and adept in language, poetry and song, this is partly a product of nineteenth-century Celtic revivalism. This revivalism was influenced by writers such as Mathew Arnold (1822–88), who contrasted the enterprising, self-reliant and self-controlled Saxon with the impulsive, child-like and mystical Celt (Ó Donnabháin 2000, 191), a construction that is embedded within the dynamics of colonialism (Nandy 1983, cited in Moane 1996). The Anglo-Irish ruling élite dominated the antiquarian studies from which the Celtic Revival in Ireland emerged. Archaeological and historical discourses from the nineteenth century have served to validate these constructions. Irish nationalism, for example, had by the nineteenth century aspirations for a united Ireland, but this was a political unity that had not existed in the past. The search for a shared glorious Celtic past shaped not only Irish nationalism but also the early years of the independent Irish Free State. The concept of this past is still retained in the public imagination, as is the idea of a 'Celtic spirituality'.

O'Loughlin (2000) argues that the need for a 'Celtic spirituality' today reflects a present-day need. Given the decline in the authority of the Catholic Church, this 'present-day need' may be a search for a replacement or a return to pre-existing materials, as Taylor states. In addition, current representations of 'Celtic spirituality' have resonances with emerging ecological, complementary health and New Age-type movements, similar to the cluster of 'alternative' social movements of which the hospice movement forms a part, as Lawton (2000) has argued.

The influence of culture

Death is a potent time at which social practices and cultural assertions can be reinforced. Taylor (1989, 179) suggests that the strong emotions released in death rituals allow the associated symbolic meaning to be particularly empowered. In Ireland, death is a central theme in much of the literature and drama of the country. The Irish wake and the practice of lamenting the dead, although not specifically Irish practices, are strong stereotypical images of Irish death rituals. Some beliefs, for instance those surrounding the Banshee, a supernatural death messenger and a uniquely Irish phenomenon, are still alive and may highlight the existence of an underlying cosmology that is different to that found in other western societies; this may form part of the cultural residue that Taylor (1995) has argued does not go away either in the society or the individual.

Traditional beliefs and practices

There are a wealth of traditions surrounding death and dying in Ireland which have been documented (O'Suilleabháin 1967; Lysaght 1995; 1996; Donnelly 1999b). Witoszek and Sheeran (1994) have argued that Irish identity is centred on a preoccupation with death. Although some traditions have died out, such as the practice of lamenting the dead, recent research by Keegan and van Doorslaer (2001) has shown that many of the traditions are valued and continue, albeit in a modified and constantly changing form. As these authors state, traditions and customs are not static; they change, some die and some become revived, such as the practice of bringing the deceased home or laying them out at home (2001, 54). New rituals are also established, such as that of personalising a religious service, although this has met with considerable resistance from the Catholic Church (Newman in *The Irish Times*, 30 March 2000). Rituals are a way of 'talking about' important issues for a culture (Sheehy 1994, 494), and the continuation of traditional rituals and the development of new ones illustrate the centrality of death within Irish culture.

Incorporating death

Witoszek and Sheeran (1994), in a study that examines Irish funerary traditions and the theme of death in Irish literature, argue that there is a preoccupation with death in Ireland. The authors consider the funerary rituals and practices as a 'Theatrum Mortis', a theatre of the dead. This way of considering the various traditions, performed by the living (the actors) for the dead (the audience), reveals an underlying cosmology that, as Witoszek and Sheeran state, is 'an acute awareness of a powerful realm bordering on the world of the living' (1994, 7).

The authors also consider that this view of the dead, one that sees the dead as occupying an almost tangible existence, is so embedded in cultural practice in Ireland that it goes unnoticed. Larkin (1999) raises this issue in his exploration of the experiences of Irish palliative care nurses, and argues that Irish society incorporates rather than denies death. In Ireland, death is present in everyday life; for instance, the practices of broadcasting death notices on local radio stations and of national newspapers announcing business closure as a mark of respect for a death are at variance with the idea of western 'death-denying societies' (1999, 125).

A distinct cosmology

There is some basis for Witoszek and Sheeran's assertion that there is a sense of a 'powerful realm bordering on the world of the living' and this may have its roots in early Irish mythology, which relates the story of three goddesses, Banba, Fodla and Eriu, in order to explain the origins of Ireland. The Celts are reputed to have encountered this triad of goddesses when they arrived in Ireland. The goddesses initially opposed their arrival, but each agreed to admit them if they would name the land after her (Green 1995). The people of the goddess, the Tuatha de Danann, were reputed to live underground and to control the fertility of the land; the Tuatha de Danann may possibly be the source of this belief in another world close to that of the living. One aspect of the goddess Eriu is as a goddess of sovereignty, and this aspect of sacred kingship is associated with the figure of the Banshee, the supernatural death messenger.

Belief in the Banshee was particularly strong from the seventeenth century until the early part of the twentieth century, a historical period associated with the extensive colonisation of Ireland by England. There is a widespread belief that the Banshee attaches herself to particular families, and that these families, whose surnames usually begin with Mac or O, are of old Irish stock (Lysaght 1995, 62). The role of the Banshee was to establish rightful ownership, legitimacy and ancestral claim to the land.

Within folklore studies the Banshee is considered as a supernatural figure with a particular function, that of sovereignty and legitimation. The social functions of ghosts and the changing nature of these over time have been documented by Finucane (1984), who maintains that from the eighteenth century onwards in England ghosts seem to lose any direct influence over family and there is a break with ancestral demands. This diminished influence was due, according to Finucane, to the gradual loss of identification with community and the extended family (*op. cit.*, 223). The reverse seems to be the case with the Banshee, however, and although the beliefs about the Banshee can be considered to be weakened (Lysaght 2001) they do represent a belief in another world in close proximity to that of the living, as

Witoszek and Sheeran maintain (1994). Lysaght argues that the belief in the Banshee is so deep-rooted in Irish culture that it will remain part of the world-view of Irish people for a long time to come (2001, 49).

Although the claims by the publishers of *Anam Cara* (1999), already referred to, bear little resemblance to historical fact, the work of poet and philosopher the late John O'Donoghue, the author of *Anam Cara*, presents eloquent reflections on death and dying. Drawing on the traditions surrounding death and dying, O'Donoghue talks about the Banshee and states that these traditions recognise that the eternal and transient worlds are 'woven in and through each other' (1999, 256). O'Donoghue also talks about the visions of deceased mothers, grandmothers and other relations, and states that 'when a person is close to death, the veil between this world and the eternal world is very thin, in some cases the veil is removed for a moment' (*op. cit.*, 256). Writing on the presence of the dead, O'Donoghue says:

> *'I feel that our friends amongst the dead really mind us and look out for us. Often there might be a big boulder of misery over your path, but your friends among the dead hold it back until you have passed by. One of the exciting developments that may happen in evolution and in human consciousness in the next several hundred years is a whole new relationship with the invisible, eternal world. We might begin to link up in a very creative way with our friends in the invisible world'* (*op. cit.*, 275).

Research on death and dying in Ireland

Recent research on palliative care and death and dying in Ireland places considerable emphasis on cultural influences. Larkin (1999) has explored, through in-depth interviews, whether being Irish is a relevant aspect in the meaning that palliative care nurses derive from their care of the dying. He established five different expressions of caring that the nurses found meaningful and which, he argues, can be considered 'Irish conceptualisations of care'. These five different expressions (*Dluchaidreamh*—closeness; *Anam chara*—soul friend; *Gramhar*—loving; *Aire*—

caring; *Spioraid*—spirit) touch on various aspects of traditional practices and beliefs and engage the language of Celtic spirituality.

Donnelly (1999b), a consultant in palliative medicine in a hospice in the mid-west of Ireland, conducted a study on the 'Folklore associated with dying in the west of Ireland', examining traditions and customs surrounding death and dying in that area. Donnelly states that while modern advances in the care for the dying are to be welcomed, care for the dying should not exclude the traditions of the past. Her study documents information from in-depth interviews conducted in rural areas in the western part of Ireland and emphasises 'the closeness of nature, expressed in the attitude to dying, reflected the life and living in these rural people and their antecedents for thousands of years' (1999b, 61).

A changing landscape

The Keegan and van Doorslaer (2001) study on attitudes to death, dying and bereavement in Ireland presents a diverse picture of contemporary Ireland. This was a qualitative study involving interviews with key informants (a palliative care educator, a funeral director, a community development worker and a psychologist specialising in bereavement work). Further focus group discussions were held with general practitioners, clergy, palliative care health professionals, teachers, community development workers and the general public.

Although the research did not specifically consider the concept of a 'good death', representations of death did emerge, with accidental death, suicides or murders and premature or untimely deaths, particularly the death of a child, considered as 'brutal' or 'tragic' (*op. cit.*, 27). On the other hand, deaths that involved a degree of preparation and the opportunity to say goodbye were felt to be more helpful for the bereaved. Deaths that occurred at the end of a long life or in a manner that was in keeping with the personality of the deceased were also considered as 'natural' (*op. cit.*, 29). These are representations of a 'good death' that fit with those discussed in the previous chapter.

The research found a changed attitude toward Catholicism, which the authors state has impacted on attitudes to death and dying—traditionally aspects of life that were very closely associated with religious practice. Some of the respondents in the study displayed a greater flexibility toward Catholic teaching and a more 'flexible Christian attitude prevailed' (2001, 17), although for most respondents a religious element in funerary rituals was important. The research also found a change in the way Irish society organises death and dying, with an emphasis more on the doctor than on the priest, and on funeral directors rather than helpful neighbours.

A shift toward individualism and away from the traditional authority of the Church, suggested by Inglis (1998), was also demonstrated in the debate concerning personal eulogies at funerals, a debate that was ongoing at the time of the Keegan and van Doorslaer (2001) study and which reflects issues of control over funeral rituals and tensions between the individual and the traditional authority of the Church.

A eulogy in remembrance of the deceased is provided for in the structure of the Mass. Traditionally this was conducted by the priest, but there is now an increasing trend toward family members conducting this. The archbishop of Armagh, Dr Seán Brady, banned eulogies by family members, claiming that eulogies did not fit with the Order of Christian Funerals— eulogies may repeat the sentiments already expressed by the priest, they may place undue stress on the person chosen to speak, and most importantly they may detract from the sacred nature of the liturgy and may be offensive to the congregation (*Irish Times*, 30 March 2000).

Walter (1990) has argued that there is an increase, in western societies, in life-centred funerals that focus on the unique personality of the deceased. The debate that took place in Ireland in 2000 may more accurately reflect a generalised trend, as objections were not confined to Catholicism. The objections to eulogies and other practices, such as choices of personal and non-religious readings and personal rather than religiously symbolic gifts being brought to the altar, raised by the Catholic Church were also supported by the Anglican Church. The dean of Christ Church, Dr Paterson, agreed with the archbishop of Armagh as 'Both churches have very fine funeral rites and there is no need to ignore them by "do-it-yourself" liturgy' (*Irish Times*, 30 March 2000).

This debate reflects issues of control over funeral rites, with, on the one hand, religious authorities wanting control over the rituals of death, and, on the other, families increasingly feeling that funerals should be more personal and relevant to them. In practice, eulogies continue to be conducted by family members, at the discretion of the local priest. These two views were reflected in the study, with some respondents expressing a wish for funerals to be more personal and others feeling that the funeral Mass was becoming too personal and losing the formal religious emphasis (Keegan and van Doorslaer 2001, 42).

The research also revealed contradictory attitudes towards traditional practices such as wakes, with some respondents feeling that these have died out and others expressing a contrary view. While it is evident from this study that a wake is the normal practice, the form that the wake takes may now be changing. The definition of a wake varied considerably—the location has become more varied, taking place in the house, pub or hotel; the timing and duration of the wake also varied, with a wake taking place either after a funeral or in the house with the corpse. Nevertheless, the emphasis on gathering and being together, with the common elements of drink and food, remained.

A central theme to emerge from the study is contradiction—on the one hand an adherence to traditional rituals and beliefs about death and dying, and, on the other, new forms of ritual and beliefs. Keegan and van Doorslaer consider that Ireland is characterised by a changing landscape—the beliefs, traditions and behaviours are changing—and in contemporary Ireland more than one explanation or guide is used as a reference for behaviour (*op cit.*, 113).

Palliative care in Ireland

With the growth of the hospice movement in the UK from the 1960s, similar developments and initiatives have taken place in Ireland. Just as the initial development of hospices in the UK took place outside of the NHS and later became incorporated within mainstream health care, a similar situation arose in Ireland.

The central position of the Catholic Church in the development and maintenance of health care has already been outlined. Hospice care in Ireland originated in the late nineteenth century with the establishment of Our Lady's Hospice in Dublin and St Patrick's Hospice in Cork by the Sisters of Charity, who have played a crucial role in the development of palliative care in Ireland (O'Brien 1995; Butler 1980); this role has also been specifically recognised by the National Advisory Committee on Palliative Care (*Report of the National Advisory Committee on Palliative Care* (RNACPC) 2001). The position of religious orders in the organisation of health care in Ireland has diminished somewhat in recent years although their ethos and vision are still quite influential (Larkin 1999), as already discussed. The current position and future development of palliative care services in Ireland need to be viewed within the context of the Irish health care service.

The Irish health service: a view from history

The Irish health care system has evolved in an ad hoc and piecemeal fashion and has been subjected to considerable influence from powerful groups, such as the medical profession and the Catholic Church, both before independence and in the early years of the new state. Prior to independence, opposition from the Catholic Church and some elements of the medical profession blocked the extension of the social insurance scheme which was introduced in the UK in 1911 (Wren 2003, 23). The establishment of a health care system on a rights basis, which led to fundamental reforms in many countries during the 1940s, for example the establishment of the NHS in the UK in 1948 and a social security system in France in 1945 (*op. cit.*, 30), was never established in Ireland, although it was attempted.

Accounts of opposition from powerful groups in medicine and the Catholic Church to progressive initiatives in the development of the health service are too numerous to document here. However, one such initiative—the Mother and Child Scheme of 1950—which met considerable opposition and ultimately failed has become a famous or rather infamous episode in Irish political and social history and is worth recounting to illustrate the degree of influence that was exercised.

The Mother and Child Scheme

In 1948 Dr Noel Browne, a medical doctor, campaigned for the provision of sanatoria for tuberculosis patients, as TB was widespread at the time in Ireland. On election he became Minister for Health and set about a radical programme of eradication of tuberculosis; he established sanatoria for the isolation and recuperation of TB patients and made these beds available irrespective of income. Between 1948 and 1953 the death rate dropped from 12.5 per 10,000 of the population in 1945 to 5.4 in 1952 (Barrington 1987). Browne had a deep personal and ideological commitment to public health, a commitment that was to cause considerable difficulties for the implementation of health care reforms.

Browne, as Minister for Health, had the task of amending the 1947 Health Act in line with concerns raised by the Catholic bishops. At this time the Catholic archbishop of Dublin, John Charles McQuaid, was a powerful force in health care; he was chairman of the largest hospital in Dublin and had control over the appointments of consultants in Catholic voluntary hospitals. McQuaid had also formed a close and politically significant bond with the Fianna Fáil leader, Éamon de Valera, which had ensured that the 1937 Constitution enshrined Catholic teaching (Cooney 1999). This Constitution strongly represents Catholic moral teaching and contained an Article that recognised 'the special position of the Holy Catholic and Apostolic and Roman Church as the guardian of the faith professed by the great majority of its Citizens'. This Article was deleted in a referendum in 1972 (Inglis 1998).

Noel Browne, although a Catholic, had undertaken his medical studies in Trinity College Dublin. McQuaid had announced in 1944 that any Catholic who attended Trinity College without his permission was guilty of a mortal sin, and until 1971 Dublin diocesan regulations continued to forbid Catholics to attend Trinity College, a Protestant institution since the sixteenth century (*ibid.*, 60). McQuaid was antagonistic toward Browne and opposed to Browne's attempts at reform, particularly the proposed changes in hospital ownership (Wren 2003, 36).

In 1950, as part of what became known as 'the Mother and Child Scheme',

Browne proposed that dispensary doctors would become district medical officers and provide free medical care for children up to sixteen years and be paid an annual amount for each patient. He also proposed free medical treatment of mothers before and after birth and for infants up to six weeks.

Browne alienated the medical profession with his proposal, although dispensary doctors stood to gain by the scheme. General practitioners, under this proposal, faced a major threat to their practice. The Irish Medical Association was alarmed by the proposals, which they saw as the first step towards the introduction of a full-time, salaried medical service under central bureaucracy, and they wrote to the Minister objecting to 'the provision of free medical treatment to non-necessitous persons' (Barrington 1987).

In addition to the opposition from the medical profession, the Catholic bishops opposed the scheme and stated, in a letter to the Taoiseach (the Irish prime minister), that the right to provide for the health of children belonged to parents, not the state. The bishops also stated that 'education in regard to motherhood includes instructions in regard to sex relations, chastity and marriage and the State had no competence in such matters'. In an apparent reference to Trinity College, the bishops' letter also stated that 'doctors trained in institutions in which we have no confidence might deliver gynaecological care which in other countries includes birth limitation and control' (Browne 1986).

In spite of opposition from the bishops and the medical profession Browne attempted to introduce his scheme, but he lost the support of the then Taoiseach, John A. Costello, who was opposed to socialised medicine and supported the bishops' arguments (*Dáil Debates*, cited in Wren 2003).

The 1953 Health Act enshrined some aspects of the Mother and Child Scheme, such as free treatment for mothers before and after the birth of a child and treatment of infants up to six weeks old. Compromises were reached with the medical profession to protect the incomes of both general practitioners and hospital consultants. In turn, a compromise was reached with the Catholic bishops that involved opening the public hospitals to clinical teaching by appointees of the university medical schools, thereby ensuring Catholic influence in the public hospitals through the medical schools of the Catholic National University (Barrington 1987).

The development of palliative care in Ireland

The diminished power of the Catholic Church has decreased its influence on the further development of the health service; however, control of some hospitals still exists, as already outlined. The original hospices established by the Sisters of Charity in Dublin and Cork became incorporated into the health service. The evolution of palliative care began, supported by the establishment of the Irish Hospice Foundation in 1986 as a voluntary support organisation for the development and improvement of hospice services. The Irish Association of Palliative Care was established in the early 1990s to promote the development of palliative care throughout Ireland. The Irish Medical Council approved the recognition of the specialism of palliative medicine in 1995.

Local and voluntary organisations have played a large part in the initial development of hospice services in Ireland, as has also been the case in the UK. Palliative care services were initially established around the country largely owing to the 'strong and concerted efforts of various voluntary organisations' (*RNACPC* 2001). The role of voluntary organisations has also been specifically recognised; in 1994 the Department of Health recognised that the voluntary sector plays 'an integral role in the provision of health and social services in Ireland which is perhaps unparalleled in any other country' (Department of Health 1994, 10).

While the role of voluntary organisations in the establishment of palliative care services is acknowledged, this has led to the ad hoc establishment of services nationwide, with a number of different and independent organisations working within each health board area. The relationships between these organisations and the health boards, in terms of reporting structure, funding and issues of responsibility, can, according to the National Advisory Committee on Palliative Care (discussed below), lead to 'unsatisfactory and often divisive relationships' (*RNACPC* 2001).

The future of palliative care in Ireland

The lack of a national policy on palliative care and the diverse range of services available around the country led the Irish Association of Palliative Care and the Irish Hospice Foundation to commission a survey of Irish palliative care services in 1993 (Igoe *et al.* 1997). All adult palliative care services (24 home care services, three in-patient services and one acute hospital service) in existence at the end of 1993 were contacted. The survey found that the palliative care service was largely a home care-based service for cancer patients (only 2% of care patients had another diagnosis). The survey also found a wide variation in staffing levels, workload, travelling, assessment of needs and finance arrangements. A major feature identified by the survey was the difficulty of providing an adequate service to a dispersed rural population, with a large difference in costs and work patterns between urban and rural services.

Arising from the 1993 survey, a position paper (Irish Association of Palliative Care and the Irish Hospice Foundation 1996) was presented to the Minister for Health. This made a number of recommendations for the future of palliative care services and addressed issues of funding, structures, standards, education and training. The establishment of a national policy for the development of services and the need for a greater partnership between the statutory and voluntary health groups involved in the provision of palliative care were also recommended.

The National Advisory Committee on Palliative Care

The Minister for Health and Children established a National Advisory Committee on Palliative Care in 1999 to report on palliative care services in Ireland. The National Advisory Committee on Palliative Care report (*RNACPC* 2001) provided a comprehensive overview of the development and level of current palliative care services and set out a number of key recommendations for the future development of services in line with developments in other countries. For instance, the committee recommended that palliative care should be structured in three levels of ascending specialisation: palliative care approach, general palliative care and specialist palliative care (a development of palliative care services outlined in the previous chapter), and that these levels of care should be available in each health board area (*op. cit.*, 32).

The demand for palliative care services is expected to rise in the coming years, in line with population growth. The number of people dying of cancer is also expected to rise owing to an ageing population. It is also proposed to extend the palliative care services to other patient groups, in line with the extension of palliative care services discussed in the previous chapter (Addington-Hall and Higginson 2001).

A number of priorities were highlighted, including the completion of needs assessment to define the palliative care needs, which in turn will inform the implementation of a national policy on palliative care. The National Advisory Committee also noted the lack of research on palliative care in Ireland and has recommended that research be undertaken, especially to evaluate the effectiveness of different models of specialist palliative care (*op. cit.*, 107).

Research in palliative care in Ireland

To date a small amount of research has been undertaken which has mainly focused on evaluation and quality-of-service issues (Igoe *et al.* 1997; Keegan *et al.* 1999). A National Needs Assessment for Paediatric Palliative Care has been undertaken in addition to an exploration of the relationship between the Travelling community and palliative care services (van Doorslaer and McQuillan 2006). Research by Larkin (1999), Donnelly (1999b), and Keegan and van Doorslaer (2001) has already been discussed.

The Keegan *et al.* (1999) study—*Care for the dying—experiences and challenges: a study of quality of health service care during the last year of life of patients at St James's Hospital, Dublin, from their relatives' perspective*—is based on the Addington-Hall and McCarthy (1995) regional study of care for the dying. The research focused on the care of patients and their families in an acute hospital, with and without the involvement of the palliative care team, and conducted structured qualitative interviews with 155 relatives.

Hospital was the location of the patient's death for 74% of the relatives in the study; 12% of patients died at home (under the care of the hospice home care team), and 14% died in a hospice. The majority of respondents felt that their relative had a 'good death'; the positive response increased, although not significantly, with palliative care involvement (1999, 9).

The research findings do not specifically define a 'good death', although it would appear to be linked to supplementary questions relating to religious and spiritual ease at the time of death and preparation for death on the part of the patient and the relatives. The results showed that 72% of those who died in the hospital without palliative care services were considered to have had a 'good death', 81% of those in the hospital with palliative care services had a 'good death', 100% of those who died in the hospice had a 'good death' and 81% of those who died at home (with the palliative care home team) had a 'good death' (*op. cit.*, 9).

The numbers relating to religious and spiritual ease show that 80% of those who died in hospital without palliative care felt at ease spiritually, 88% of those who died in hospital with palliative care felt at ease, while 86% of hospice patients and 86% of those who died at home experienced religious and spiritual ease.

The research also focused on aspects of palliative care such as communication and breaking bad news, and suggests that when palliative care principles were adhered to—in relation to good communication, spending time, breaking bad news gently but clearly—the relatives appreciated this approach. The research also documented many instances where patients were told bad news alone with no family or social support; some relatives were told in corridors, and one person was told over the telephone (*op. cit.*, 13). The research found that the hospital doctor was most frequently the person who broke bad news, and results showed that relatives were told by the doctor while the patient may not have been. Some relatives found this difficult, finding it stressful that there was uncertainty concerning awareness of the prognosis by the patient. This difficulty also meant that any talk about death between relatives and patients was unlikely. At the same time most relatives did not talk to their family member about the possibility of death and remained glad of this fact.

Patients who received palliative care were more likely to have been informed directly of their diagnosis (*op. cit.*, 62).

An aspect of communication highlighted in the report was the failure to notify relatives of deterioration, and the research found that there was considerable dissatisfaction with this aspect of hospital care. Relatives also expressed considerable dissatisfaction with procedures concerning admission to hospital, with long waiting times in accident and emergency, repetition of questions about their medical illness and history, and their uncertainty about what was going on (*op. cit.*, 63). Patients in the Young and Cullen (1996) study, discussed in the previous chapter, made similar comments about difficulties in attending hospital.

The majority of respondents in the study had a positive view of the care received in the hospital. The authors suggest that the presence of a palliative care team in an acute hospital may have promoted a palliative care approach, with the key principles of sensitivity, respect, regard for patient choice, provision of information and care for the family being demonstrated in most instances (*op. cit.*, 59).

The research made a number of key recommendations—a need for specific training in communication and for the formal assignment of responsibility for informing patients about their diagnosis. It was also recommended that patients with advanced and progressive illness should have immediate access to care through accident and emergency departments, while at the same time avoiding a repetition of questions relating to illness and medical history. The research also recommended that future research on the current context of, and attitude to, death in Ireland would serve as a baseline to evaluate change in perceived quality of clinical care, the attitudes of health professionals, and the expectations and attitudes of the Irish population regarding death (*op. cit.*, 66).

A perspective on healing

Barthes (1993, 109) has argued that myth is a 'form of speech, it is a system of communication', and it is clear from the previous discussions that the discourse on a 'Celtic spirituality', beliefs in the supernatural figure of the Banshee and all she signifies, and the focus of the research work of Larkin (1999) and Donnelly (1999b) draw considerably on a mythic past in order to make sense of the present.

The work of Dr Michael Kearney, which has been influential in both Irish palliative care and the international palliative care community, also draws on mythology but in this case it is Greek mythology. In two reflective publications, *Mortally wounded* (1996) and *A place of healing: working with suffering in living and dying* (2000), Kearney has explored the nature of soul pain and healing. Based on his experience of caring for dying people—Dr Kearney was a consultant in palliative medicine in Dublin and also trained and worked at St Christopher's Hospice in London—he examines the nature of both the surface and the depth work that he considers to be part of palliative care.

Kearney's understanding of suffering and the resolution of suffering has roots in antiquity, in early shamanism and in the Greek mythological story of Chiron—the wounded healer. Kearney views the wounded healer as a mythological way of understanding both the nature of distress and ways in which the individual might move beyond suffering to a place of healing (1996, 42). He has taken the idea of 'total pain', discussed in the previous chapter, and developed the aspect of soul pain; his approach is independent of religious doctrine and has been developed from secular psychological models. Nevertheless, his work reflects attributes of spiritual care advocated by Saunders (1965; 1988) and Stanworth (1997), i.e. the emphasis on metaphor and symbolism, as discussed in the previous chapter.

Kearney explains that Chiron, a centaur, was born of a god and a human, and was half mortal, half immortal. Abandoned and rejected at birth, he was adopted by the sun-god Apollo. He became a wise and respected teacher. Chiron was wounded with a poisoned arrow which, as he was half immortal, did not kill him but inflicted an agonising and unhealable wound. He withdrew to the mountains to tend to his wound and began a search to release him from his suffering, a search which lasted the rest of his life. Although he did not find his own cure, he became wise in the use of all healing herbs and compassionate to the sufferings of others. He became known as the 'wounded healer'. Chiron was granted freedom from his suffering if he sacrificed his immortality. He agreed to this, died and descended to the underworld. For nine days and nights he remained in the darkness of death. Zeus, acknowledging his sacrifice, restored his immortality, raising him to the heavens as a constellation of stars.

Chiron's behaviour in this myth is determined, according to Kearney, by two radically different viewpoints. The first—a heroic stance— is evident in the first part of his life as he struggled to overcome his adversity. A key moment comes when he chooses to let go of his immortality, and from then on his actions come from a different viewpoint, 'the way of descent'. This turning point 'marks a transition from one realm to another, from the above to the below, from the known to the unknown' (Kearney 1996, 43–4).

Kearney argues that moving from the surface to the deep mind is the same psychological process involved in Chiron's change from a heroic stance to the way of descent. This is a pivotal shift in the dying process, according to Kearney, and this downward shift happens naturally, quietly and invisibly for most people in their own time and enables individuals to experience a new peace, richness and 'a depth in their living and their dying' (1996, 60).

For some people this process does not occur and they remain trapped at the surface level of their mind, 'cut off from the healing power of their own inner depths' (*op. cit.*, 60). These people can exhibit tremendous suffering prior to death, and Kearney describes, through a series of case-studies, ways in which interventions such as image-work, dream-work, art and other therapies have enabled the individual to move into depth and thus beyond suffering (*op. cit.*, 65).

Kearney developed and expanded his understanding of healing as an innate ability in his more recent publication, *A place of healing* (2000). In this he states more forcibly the basic assumption that underlies his work—that in working with suffering, healing is something that happens rather than something that is done. He considers the role of those working with dying people to be to help create the environment where what is 'fundamental, natural and indigenous in the human psyche can most easily do its own work in bringing about integration, balance and wholeness' (2000, xxii).

Kearney expands on his previous work and returns to Greek mythology in an attempt to overcome the limitations of the medical model in addressing the suffering of individuals. The underworld or 'chthonic' god Asklepios exercised healing through an alliance with nature and the powers of the earth and, according to Kearney, Asklepian healing is not found in the surface mind but in the deep, quantum realms of the body and soul (2000, 65). There are two principles of Asklepian healing: the way through 'soul sickness'—that is, suffering is found within the depths of the person who suffers—and healing is dependent on an encounter with the 'divine'. Healing comes through an encounter with some autonomous element within the depths of that person; 'there is a journey inwards and there is waiting' (*op. cit.*, 67).

Kearney acknowledges the strengths of the medical model in easing the pain of terminal illness but argues that there are limitations to the alleviation of suffering that are inherent in this model. Kearney returns to the roots of the medical model and draws threads of connection between, as he sees it, the twin strands of Hippocratic medicine and Asklepian healing, one which works to treat pain and lessen the suffering by intervening from outside the person (Hippocratic) and the other (Asklepian) concerned with the healing of suffering from within (*op. cit.*, 37). Kearney advocates an integration of Hippocratic and Asklepian models in a new model of health care.

Kearney's proposed integrated model of health care is a further development of the palliative care model that draws on a secular rather than a Christian ideal of care. In drawing, however, on the mythological stories of ancient Greece, he uses the same form of language a symbolic language—that is present in conceptualisations of 'Celtic spirituality', Catholicism and the spirituality discourse expounded by Stanworth (1997) and Czechmeister (1994).

Summary

This chapter set out to consider the degree to which the 'manner of parting' may have been shaped by culture in Ireland. It is clear that the Catholic Church in Ireland has been a powerful influence in all aspects of Irish society, although its power has declined since the 1970s with a marked decrease in vocations in addition to factors of modernisation and the impact of sexual and child abuse scandals.

A new type of Catholic is emerging—Protestant Catholics, who no longer look to the Church for religious authority—along with a belief in a spirit or life force rather than a personal God. Disillusionment with the Church and a more individual approach to religious or spiritual belief may be reflected in the popularity of 'Celtic spirituality', which draws on a mythic past.

Little research has been conducted on death and dying in Ireland, and no study has specifically considered the concept of a 'good death'. Implicit understandings of a 'good death' include preparation, saying goodbye and being at religious and spiritual ease. An integrated model of health care, incorporating healing and medical models, has been advocated, based on the understanding that healing is an innate ability in all individuals and that health care needs to provide the right environment for this to occur. This new model also draws on mythology, using a form of symbolic language that is compatible with other discourses, such as those of religion and spirituality.

Strong traditions, beliefs and rituals around death and dying in Ireland have led some commentators to argue that death plays a central role in Irish life. It has also been argued that a different cosmology exists in Ireland, one that sees and experiences a powerful realm bordering on the world of the living. Recent research suggests that Ireland is characterised by a changing landscape—the beliefs, traditions and behaviours are changing—and that in contemporary Ireland more than one explanation or guide is used as a reference. Nevertheless, these explanations appear, as yet, to be conducted through symbolic or religious language and understandings.

CHAPTER 3
The means of exploration

Introduction

This book is based on an ethnographic study within a hospice in Ireland that used a grounded theory approach and qualitative methods of observation and in-depth interviews. The conceptual framework that guided the research was one of exploration and cartography. This chapter describes preliminary research, the conceptual framework and the research design, the research methods of ethnography and grounded theory, ethical considerations, data collection and methods of analysis.

Preliminary research

The aims and focus of the research may appear as ready-formulated questions but research does not always proceed in an orderly fashion. Rock (2001) argues that research is not passive or neutral but interactive and creative, selective and interpretative, with further paths of enquiry opening up as the work progresses. Research is a process that changes with each stage of the enquiry, and many important questions emerge only *in situ* (2001, 30).

The original focus of this research concerned the phenomenon of Nearing Death Awareness (NDA). NDA was identified by two US hospice nurses, Callanan and Keeley (1997), and is used to describe a phenomenon whereby some dying people develop an awareness of when they are going to die and experience visions of those already deceased. This term was first used by Callanan and Keeley and is based on their own and other nurses' experiences of dying patients.

Deathbed visions have been documented throughout history and across cultures (Barrett 1926; Zaleski 1987; Basford 1990). An early reference appears in *The cyclopaedia of anatomy and physiology* (1836). Physician J. A. Symonds, in the course of writing about the medical indicators of death, describes the deathbed visions of some of his patients. He speculates that:

> *'the spectra owe their origin to contemplations of future existence; and consequently that the good man's last hours are cheered with beatific visions and communion with heavenly visitors'* (Basford 1990, 131).

According to Callanan and Keeley (1997), part of the difficulty in researching the experiences of dying people is that they may be expressed through symbolic language or gesture and this form of communication does not lend itself easily to scientific enquiry, which may have contributed to these experiences being overlooked in the past. The original research focus sought to explore how these experiences, as documented by Callanan and Keeley, were understood from different perspectives, such as those of family members, nursing staff and chaplains.

I conducted a number of pilot interviews, using a snowballing recruitment method (Bowling 1997; Arksey and Knight 1999). It became apparent, however, from these pilot interviews that aspects of NDA, such as perceiving the presence of deceased relatives, were understood within the context of a 'good death'. Deathbed visions certainly did occur: for instance, one participant related to me that as her mother-in-law was dying she saw her previously deceased son (the participant's husband) and this gave her mother-in-law great consolation and peace. What was important to the participant was the outcome, peace and consolation, not the vision itself. Continuing to pursue accounts of deathbed visions and other aspects of NDA would, I felt, have resulted in a 'list', and one that prompted further questions which seemed to be concerned with understandings of a 'good death'. Questions about a 'good death' also prompt questions about how this may be culturally shaped. As a result of the pilot interviews, this research came to focus on the more fundamental question of how a 'good death' was understood and defined in Ireland.

Changing direction

The findings of the pilot study changed the direction of the research toward an exploration of the concept of a 'good death'. Rock (2001, 33) suggests that it is 'prudent to search for a problem that is an extension of the known, a logical next step from territory that is familiar'. While Rock advocates this as a mechanism for combating intellectual solitude, it emerged from the pilot study that NDA is not a familiar experience for many people and it seemed prudent, therefore, to research a more general concept before embarking on any research concerning deathbed visions or other aspects of NDA.

The opportunity to focus on the concept of a 'good death' rather than NDA came about in a fashion that Fetterman (1989, 12) has suggested is one of the hallmarks of ethnography—that is, a mixture of 'serendipity, creativity, being in the right place at the right or wrong time and old fashioned luck'. A number of factors converged to shift the direction. The snowballing method of recruitment of participants for pilot interviews was becoming inadequate for the purpose; it was unreliable for recruiting sufficient numbers of people within the time-frame and there was an inbuilt bias towards recruitment of like-minded people, which can be a difficulty with this method (Arksey and Knight 1999). At this point the old-fashioned luck that Fetterman describes came into play. Contact was made with a doctor working in palliative care who was interested in researching how patients, family members and professional staff defined a 'good death' and this shifted the direction of the research toward palliative care and a focus on a 'good death' and spiritual care.

Conceptual framework

The shift to an exploration of a 'good death' and spiritual care within a palliative care setting demanded a re-evaluation of the research methods. Focusing on palliative care and the population of people within palliative care settings—patients, family members, professional and non-professional staff and volunteers—overcame the recruitment difficulties experienced during the preliminary research. However, involvement in the social world of a palliative care setting presented other research challenges.

A focus on palliative care, the central tenet of which is the facilitation of a 'good death', as discussed in Chapter 1, provided the opportunity to explore this question with people who, to varying degrees, focused on the experiences of death and dying. A 'good death' within palliative care may have its own internal values and logic, however, and some method of understanding these values and this social world was necessary. Within this framework, the role of the researcher can more clearly be seen as that of a visitor in the social world of the participants in the research and the hospice itself.

Viewing the role of the researcher as visitor highlighted the dynamics involved in entering into other social worlds—that of the hospice and the participants—and the consequent responsibilities or ethical considerations. The degree to which the researcher can become assimilated into these worlds, becoming part of the 'family' and less of a visitor in a sense, depends on the degree of trust and intimacy that develops, and these are important aspects of qualitative research. The researcher, as visitor, also requires a map of these social worlds and the research process can be considered as akin to a cartographic exercise: the research is the creation of a map. Mapping, maps and the researcher as visiting cartographer not only provide useful metaphors for the research and the research process but also operate as a useful organising principle for the various strands of this research.

Cartography

Elias has stated that, apart from religious death rituals, dying 'is at present a largely unformed situation, a blank area on the social map' (1985, 28). Harley (1988) has likened cartography to a 'form of knowledge and a form of power'; who draws the map and what is documented as important features are critical questions. Drawing on the work of Foucault, he asserts that the knowledge and production of cartography is a 'way of presenting one's own values in the guise of scientific disinterestedness' (1988, 279). His discussion of maps—the way in which power structures the content of maps and how cartographic communication on a symbolic level can reinforce these power structures through map knowledge (1988, 280)—has a resonance with the biomedical model and theories of death, dying and bereavement.

As already discussed in Chapter 1, the palliative care model is a person-focused approach to care. It also raises a question, however, as to whether this model accurately reflects the phenomenological world of the patients and their families or whether the surveying tools of the biomedical model have been more skilfully and rigorously applied, as Arney and Bergen (1984) and Clark's (1999) arguments imply. There are a number of themes that can usefully be served by the image of maps and cartography. The dynamics of colonialism and imperialism can be revealed in the strategies of mapping. These include 'the reinscription, enclosure and hierarchisation of space' (Blunt and Rose 1994, 10), which has parallels with the incorporation and legitimating process at work within medical models of care such as the incorporation of the hospice model of care as a biomedical specialism.

Social maps

Creating maps that chart the social space occupied by the participants within their social and political contexts and over time may begin to set in motion what Lefebvre considers a 'specific dialectic' in which 'a unity transpires between levels which analysis keeps separate from one another' (1991, 85). The idea of social space as conceptualised by Lefebvre is very wide-ranging; the space occupied by a social group or several groups is not fixed. Spaces can be combined or superimposed and may even sometimes collide (*ibid.*, 86). The language and discourse that emanate from these spaces, the verbal and non-verbal signs, potentially enhance the accuracy of these maps.

Each of the aspects of this research—the culture of palliative care, team working and professional roles, relationship and place, spiritual care and a 'good death'—can be considered as maps in themselves, maps that are interwoven and overlapping, and are set out as such in the following chapters. The individual maps of the participants in the research can be drafted onto these maps; through fitting them together to see more clearly where they merge, connect or even collide, to borrow Lefebvre's phrase, a multi-dimensional map may emerge.

Research design

Ethnography involves an emphasis on discovery and understanding. As this research focused on a particular aspect of palliative care, some mechanism for sharpening the focus on understandings of a 'good death' and spiritual care was needed in order to complement rather than conflict with the ethnographic approach. Charmaz and Mitchell (2001, 160) advocate the use of grounded theory methods and approach to help ethnographers conduct efficient fieldwork and create astute analysis as both share common roots within symbolic interactionism, and although they have developed differently the two approaches can complement each other. According to Charmaz and Mitchell,

> *'using grounded theory methods can streamline fieldwork and move ethnographic research toward theoretical interpretation. Attending to ethnographic methods can prevent grounded theory studies from dissolving into quick and dirty qualitative research'* (2001, 60).

While researchers such as Charmaz and Mitchell argue that grounded theory can sharpen the focus of ethnography, an ethnographic study with a physical presence in the research field and attention paid to the physical space and materials of the research area, in addition to interview data, is also advocated by Sandelowski, who argues that the 'ground in grounded theory is also a material/physical place/space' (2002, 112).

Ethnography

The underlying rationale of ethnography is that society and culture can only be studied from the inside by immersion of the researcher in the society under study, and it relies upon the researcher, through the process of observation, as the primary research instrument (Walsh 2001, 218). This view stands in contrast to a positivist view of social phenomena that emphasises neutrality and objectivity (*ibid.*, 217). Rock (2001) has described ethnography as a loose term that covers situated, empirical description of people and races. Research methods used as part of ethnographic research include fieldwork, participant observation and other qualitative research methods. This variety of sources for the collection of data may be utilised in order to arrive at what Geertz (1973) has termed 'thick description', i.e. the multi-layered meanings that are present in any social action. As such, ethnography is an appropriate approach when cultural attributes are specifically under study, as cultural beliefs and values are embodied within and through social action.

Grounded theory

Grounded theory has its origins in the symbolic interactionist perspective developed by G. H. Mead (1934). Two variants of symbolic interactionism developed from Mead's work, one based at the University of Chicago. The Chicago School emphasised the more involved role of the social researcher, with a central goal being the empathic understanding of the subject under research. A focus on the social meanings that emerge develops understanding and consequently affects the behaviour of those involved (Layder 1993). This approach to social research utilises methods that facilitate exploration of meanings, such as observation, in-depth and semi-structured interviews and documentary evidence. Hammersley has argued that the main assumption underlying qualitative research methods is that 'the social world must be discovered and this can only be achieved through first-hand observation and participation in "natural" settings and guided by an exploratory orientation' (1990, 598).

Grounded theory was developed by Glaser and Strauss through their research into the hospital care of dying patients (1965). It arose from their dissatisfaction with sociological theorising that seemed generally speculative in nature as it had not grown directly out of research. As a result, it did not 'fit' the real world and held little relevance to the people concerned (Layder 1993). Glaser and Strauss state that, whether or not there is a previous speculative theory, discovery 'gives us a theory that "fits or works" since the theory has been derived from data, not deduced from logical assumptions' (1967, 30).

While Glaser and Strauss formulated grounded theory in order to arrive at formal theory, there are preliminary stages to the generation of formal theory. They state that 'many ethnographic studies and multiple theories are needed so that various substantive and formal areas of inquiry can continue to build up to more inclusive formal theories' (1967, 35).

The process by which substantive theory may be formulated is through generating hypotheses that require only enough evidence to establish a suggestion. Glaser and Strauss state that in the beginning these hypotheses may seem unrelated, but as categories and properties emerge, develop in abstraction and become related, their accumulating interrelation forms an integrated theoretical framework—the core of the emerging theory. The core then becomes a theoretical guide to the further collection and analysis of data (1967, 40).

Grounded theory does not impose a theoretical model on the data but allows the overall pertinent themes to emerge as the data are collected. This process identifies when new themes or issues cease to occur and therefore when sufficient data have been collected. In this way grounded theory can be considered as the sheet on which the map is drawn—as data are collected the salient features emerge. The preliminary review of the literature, presented in the previous chapters, forms the outline of the map, the state of knowledge of what is already known before the new or amended maps are drawn.

Ethical considerations

There are general principles that guide the conduct of any research. These can be considered in terms of duty toward participants and protection of the rights of participants (Murphy and Dingwall 2001). These principles have been stated as: non-maleficence—that researchers should avoid harming participants; beneficence—that research with humans should produce some positive and identifiable benefit and not be carried out simply for its own sake; autonomy—that the values of research participants should be respected; and justice—that all participants should be treated equally (Beauchamp *et al.* 1982).

These guiding principles apply irrespective of whether qualitative or quantitative methods are used. Nevertheless, the practice of these principles can be complex in conducting qualitative research. Murphy and Dingwall (2001) have specifically addressed the practice of these ethical considerations in ethnography. They argue that while the risks associated with ethnographic research are not of the same order as, for instance, biomedical research and administration of drugs or new treatments, ethnographic research is not risk-free and its potential for harm should not be lightly dismissed (*op. cit.*, 340).

The ethical principles of non-maleficence, beneficence, autonomy and justice can be directly applied in qualitative research to issues of informed consent, the right to privacy and protection from harm, which are the ethical concerns that social researchers have traditionally addressed (Denzin and Lincoln 2003, 89).

Informed consent

Underlying the principle of informed consent are two issues: that individuals are competent to make rational and mature decisions and that their agreement to participate in the research is given voluntarily (Homan 1991).

In order to make rational and mature decisions individuals need to be given sufficient information; however, Arksey and Knight (1999, 133) state that it is important to strike a balance between over- and under-informing people. It is important not to make the process too complicated by going into too much detail, although fuller information needs to be provided for qualitative in-depth interviews which are more likely to touch on sensitive issues. Information for potential participants needs to ensure that people are informed of the purpose and nature of the study, the anticipated benefits, the contact details of the researcher and the research base, the type of questions being asked and how long the interview should take. Potential participants also need to be assured that they have a right not to answer questions and to change their mind and withdraw from the research. Statements concerning anonymity and confidentiality need to state what information will be disclosed, for what purpose and to whom, and how quotations will be utilised (*ibid.*, 133).

Informed consent is a mechanism for showing respect for the rights and welfare of research participants, but it also shifts some of the responsibility from the researcher to the participant, and demonstrates that the researcher's responsibilities have been discharged and that potential harm and discomfort have been explained. This process also transforms participants from passive objects into active subjects (Alderson 1995).

The right to privacy

The right to privacy encompasses the central issue of confidentiality. Confidentiality is about not disclosing the identity of the research participants and not attributing comments to individuals in ways that can identify the individuals and institutions with which they are associated (Arksey and Knight 1999, 132). All reasonable efforts should be undertaken to preserve anonymity, such as using code numbers for interview transcripts or by assigning interviewees different names and disguising the location of the study by using a fictitious name (*ibid.*, 134).

It is, however, difficult to completely ensure confidentiality in ethnographic studies as these are generally carried out in a single research setting or a small number of settings (Murphy and Dingwall 2001). Seymour and Ingleton highlight difficulties in trying to achieve a 'thick description' that relies heavily on 'natural language and direct quotes', which means that individual anonymity can be difficult to uphold (1999, 71). Particular difficulties may arise in small departments in some organisations, such as in the Burgess study (1985, cited in Murphy and Dingwall 2001) of a comprehensive school that focused on one department comprised of only four members of staff. In this case the use of pseudonyms was not completely effective in disguising individuals. Murphy and Dingwall (2001, 341) state that ethnographers are rarely able to give absolute guarantees that the identities of people and places will remain hidden.

Protection from harm

Participating in research is not a neutral experience, and while it may not be a negative one it can raise uncomfortable questions and issues. In-depth interviews aim to go beneath superficial responses to obtain meanings that individuals assign to events and the complexities of their attitudes, behaviours and experiences (Bowling 1997, 336). Interviews are also a way to access the perspective of the person being interviewed and to find out from them things that cannot be directly observed (Patton 1990), and can facilitate the exploration of the meaning of individual experience.

Payne (1997) has stated that many people find it flattering to have the opportunity to talk about themselves and to have the attention of a researcher, and interviews can be a positive experience for both interviewer and interviewee. There are also potential benefits for participants who take part in interviews: contributing to research can be gratifying and may increase confidence, and people's own knowledge may increase (Arksey and Knight 1999, 127). There is also potential for harm, however. Interviews can involve intrusion into people's private and personal spheres and may cause embarrassment, distress and nervous strain (*ibid.*, 127).

Arksey and Knight have outlined a guide to good practice when asking sensitive questions in qualitative interviews. They state that interviewers need to be sensitive to the needs of interviewees and to let the interviewee lead in choosing whether to introduce especially distressing issues or when to draw back. Interviewers need to listen, be supportive and encouraging, and empathise with the interviewee. These guidelines for good practice also state that interviews should end on a positive note and, if appropriate, information concerning local agencies to approach for guidance, support and help may be offered (*op. cit.*, 113).

Ethical considerations in palliative care research

The need for research and critical evaluation was recognised at the foundation of the modern hospice movement. The main aim of research in palliative care is to identify ways in which the quality of life for patients and their families may be improved (Richards *et al.* 1998, 399). Understanding the experiences of dying people and those who care for them is important in an effort to improve care. Randall and Downie (1996) have stated that all kinds of research involving human subjects are likely to raise ethical problems but that research in the palliative care field is especially sensitive.

Interviewing terminally ill patients

One aspect of research within palliative care that raises particular ethical problems concerns interviewing patients or their relatives as, according to Randall and Downie (1996, 175), it is easy to fall into the trap of thinking that only invasive or drug-related care raises serious ethical problems. Nevertheless, the literature on ethical considerations regarding patient interviews contains compelling arguments for interviewing dying patients. Kellehear (1989, 65) argues that:

> *'there is certainly a case that without information and without questioning there is only speculation and opinion and without information about what may be typical or normal, people may feel their own experiences are unusual or deviant'.*

A central ethical question in palliative care is whether it is fair to expect people who are terminally ill to give up their valuable time for research. Many researchers have stated that there have been enough studies based on interviewing dying patients to discount a view that these patients should not be interviewed at all. David Field (1995) cites considerable evidence for this view: Hinton 1980; McDonnell 1989; Cartwright and Seale 1990; Higginson *et al.* 1990; Kellehear 1990; Dand *et al.* 1991; Field *et al.* 1993; Spillar and Alexander 1993; and Townsend 1993. Research has shown that dying people welcome the opportunity to tell their own story, even if this is difficult, uncomfortable or painful (Kellehear 1989), although Kellehear (1998, 72) has also argued that research is always about 'interfering with people' and the responsibility for researchers is to minimise this disturbance. The ethical task for researchers is to enable these voices to be heard in a way that causes the least intrusion.

There is also the issue of what kind of questions can be asked of dying patients and when these can be asked. Louise de Raeve wrote what she called a 'provocative' article on the ethical issues in palliative care research from a concern that there was inadequate moral scrutiny of the research process in palliative care (1994, 302). De Raeve questions whether the researcher and the dying person are coming from two different perspectives which are not necessarily compatible; the dying person, in the process of dying, may be slowly disengaging from the world, 'whereas a research enquiry seems to require the opposite: that people remain engaged and do not "slip away"' (*op. cit.*, 302). De Raeve also argues that there may be questions that are always fundamentally unanswerable and some questions about death and the process of dying may be among them. She states that perhaps the only respectful position is to 'simply and gratefully receive what is generously and spontaneously offered' (*op. cit.*, 302).

De Raeve's views elicited a strong response from leading palliative care practitioners (Mount *et al.* 1995), who took issue with many of the points she raised, including her distinction between the living and the dying. Mount *et al.* state that 'the terminally ill are living', and also argue that de Raeve's suggestion that terminally ill patients be disqualified as research participants owing to their frailty is demeaning and unacceptable and suggests that they are no longer capable of autonomous decision-making, participating in society, giving to others or finding meaning and purpose (1995, 165).

Ethical decision-making

The ethical guidelines outlined in the social research literature present fundamental ethical standards for the protection of participants that must be observed if ethical research is to be undertaken. Much, however, of the ethical decision-making in social research takes place in an ongoing and changing set of circumstances long after approval has been received from ethics committees.

Kellehear has argued that only so much basic work can be achieved by theoretical discussion of methods and ethics and that the most relevant and practical approaches come from actual work-in-progress (1989, 71). Other researchers, such as Davies and Dodd (2003, 281), offer similar reflections and perceive ethics to be always in progress, never to be taken for granted, flexible and responsive to change. Davies and Dodd advocate an understanding of ethics that involves an ongoing process of truthfulness, openness, honesty, respectfulness and constant attentiveness in order for ethics to become more than a form that is filled out for ethics committees.

Seymour and Ingleton (1999), in a discussion of ethical issues in qualitative research at the end of life, also view ethical behaviour as a practical dynamic and interpersonal activity. This activity depends on striking a balance between the rights of the individual participants, the risks of exploitation and the wider purposes of the research. They suggest that while these are relevant issues for all qualitative research, they are particularly relevant in research that involves sensitive subjects and potentially vulnerable subjects (1999, 72).

Kellehear (1989) argues that guidelines issued by professional associations and bodies serve as important points of reference for the ethical dilemmas which can arise in practical research work, but ethical conduct derives from a way of seeing and interpreting relationships and these guidelines can never encompass the diversity and complexity of each social setting. The most responsible ethics, according to Kellehear, will be those that arise from the particular social and moral complexities of the research, the particular characteristics of participants, and their social and political contexts (1989, 72).

Methodology for this study

Access to minority communities or specialist organisations can be difficult, and if research is to be conducted in an organisation it is important to start at the top and work downwards (Arksey and Knight 1999, 123). The change in focus of this research was assisted by the fortuitous meeting of a palliative care health professional interested in exploring the concept of a 'good death', as already discussed. As a result I developed a research proposal and met with a consultant in palliative medicine in the location where the research subsequently took place. Permission to undertake the research that would include in-depth interviews with a variety of staff in the hospice in addition to family members and terminally ill patients was granted.

Establishing trustworthiness is an essential part of any social research but particularly so in sensitive research areas, such as end-of-life care. The professional staff have a duty of care to patients and their families but can also be protective of them. I had preliminary meetings with key organisational personnel, including the line managers from the various departments in the hospice, which provided an opportunity to develop an overall sense of how the organisation fitted together and a strategy for recruiting interviewees from each of the departments. Those I spoke with became very committed to the research, demonstrated by helpful suggestions for contacting members of staff, the provision of staff lists in order for me to write to people individually, and facilitating staff attendance at meetings.

These meetings, and the informal chats that often followed, provided additional information about the views people held that may not otherwise have been immediately apparent. For instance, following a meeting with the day care manager to discuss the research and what was involved, I sat and chatted informally over a cup of tea with the staff of the day care centre. When I mentioned that I might like to talk to day care patients, some of the day care staff expressed a reluctance to include day care patients in the study and felt that their inclusion reflected a general view that day care patients were 'not really ill', a view they did not share. A change in management in the day centre occurred during my fieldwork and the new manager was keen for day care patients to be included.

Approximately ten weeks from the onset of the research I was allocated desk and office space close to the in-patient unit. This office space was shared with some administration staff and one volunteer and provided me with a more 'permanent' status in the organisation.

Triangulation

The idea of triangulation derives from surveying and navigation, in which people discover their position on a map by taking bearings on two landmarks, lines from which will intersect at the observer's position (Seale 1990, 54). Denzin (1970) has outlined methodological triangulation, and Hammersley and Atkinson describe it as a method whereby 'links between concepts and indictors are checked by recourse to other indicators' (1983, 199).

In this research the combination of field notes, observation and interviews created a triangulating process by which data could be verified. In addition, a form of triangulation was adopted in the creation of exploratory questions for the interviews from the theoretical model of spiritual care as proposed by Kellehear (2000b) (and discussed in Chapter 1). The contexts that Kellehear outlined in his model—situational needs, social or biographical needs and religious needs—were taken as a basis for exploratory questions.

Observation

The initial weeks of the on-site research involved preliminary meetings with key members of staff, and time spent in the hospice waiting for and having meetings facilitated the observation of the activity and daily life in the hospice. Two areas provided opportunities for observation and generally 'hanging about'. One place was a couch in the main reception area. This area was where people entered and left the hospice but also served as a central gateway to the home care offices and to the in-patient unit. There was a lot of activity here, with staff and patients and their families, and frequently members of the public who came into the hospice to hand over monies from fund-raising activities. The canteen frequented by staff, volunteers, family members and occasionally patients served as another location for 'hanging about'. Both areas provided an opportunity to become familiar with the hospice and the way in which people interacted, and for me to become a familiar face around the hospice.

Field diary and notes

Field diaries are always advocated in ethnography (Howarth 1993). Field diaries were begun at the onset of the preliminary research and provided a way to keep track of my own thinking and reflections. Looking back to the time of the preliminary research, my notes record a growing sense of 'losing the plot'—that the initial research focus was not really the fundamental question. A research diary continued throughout and, in addition to providing a record of what was happening, the diary recorded my own emotional highs and lows and anxieties relating to the research, and especially my unease about interviewing patients.

Interviewing

Interviewing can be a powerful way to assist people in making explicit their perceptions and understandings, which up to the time of interviewing may have been implicit (Arksey and Knight 1999, 32). Interviewing is a social interaction and as such is a shared communication (Davies and Dodd 2003). It is also a way to access the perspective of the person being interviewed and to find out from them things we cannot directly observe (Patton 1990) and facilitates exploration of the meaning of individual experience. Payne (1997) has advocated in-depth interviewing as the most appropriate method when the well-being of patients is paramount and thus it is the most appropriate way of exploring meaning with people in a palliative care setting.

Profile of participants

An invitation to participate in the study was issued to all staff. A total of 47 interviews were conducted and ranged in duration from 35 minutes to 90 minutes, the average being 75 minutes. Interviews were conducted with administration staff (7), volunteers (6), kitchen staff (2), care assistants (2), nurses (18), doctors (4), social workers (3), chaplains (4) and one patient. Some of those I interviewed had experience of family members dying in either a hospice, including the hospice where the research took place, or an acute hospital. All names have been changed, and in some cases the gender of the participants has been changed. The position held in the organisation has not been changed in order to retain the perspective from which participants are speaking. In some cases, the views of participants have been labelled as 'family member'; many staff spoke from a dual perspective of family member and member of staff.

Formulating questions

The formulation of questions for the interviews was based on Kellehear's (2000b) theoretical model of spiritual care (discussed in Chapter 1). The intention was to provide, in the interview questions, a set of theoretical 'fixed points' based on Kellehear's model of spiritual needs in the context of palliative care.

Kellehear's model proposed a number of dimensions to the social and spiritual aspects of care. I considered these as broad themes—social, biographical and religious aspects of needs—and devised a small number of questions in relation to each of these dimensions. For instance, for patients and family members the proposed focus was on what and who give comfort in the home, work and social aspects, and also in relation to the religious needs. Questions concerning how these aspects can be talked about and with whom also formed part of the interview schedule. In a similar way, the questions devised for the professional staff in the hospice were intended to draw on their observations of who and what can provide comfort and how this can be understood. The interview questions also focused on a personal understanding of a good death and spiritual care.

Interview format

In addition to the interview questions already described, the interview schedule included opening questions for each participant concerning how they came to work in the hospice. This first question was designed to open up the interview in a conversational manner and to act as an 'ice-breaker' but became more important than had originally been anticipated. For many of the administration staff, their initial contact with the hospice had begun with the death of a close relative in this palliative care service. The opening question in these cases moved the conversation quite smoothly into what became family members' accounts. Their subsequent working relationship with the hospice did not arise directly from the relationship of care, but frequently a couple of years later. Some of the participants had maintained a connection with the hospice and were aware of when job vacancies arose.

For many of the nursing staff and medical staff, the move to working in palliative care arose from frustration and dissatisfaction in mainstream health care settings, although for some staff a personal experience with palliative care services through the death of a family member was also a motivating factor. In relating the frustration of working in other health care settings, the course of the interview flowed easily into aspects of palliative care that were different from the curative model utilised in the hospital setting. Relating their career history, many of the professional staff talked about differences within the service, for instance between the in-patient unit and home care.

Impact of the research

The impact of the research on the researcher is part and parcel of the research process, although infrequently referred to in the research literature. One aspect of this is the complicated role of the researcher and raises questions about the nature of the role—is it that of a detached researcher, counsellor, confessor or friend? Howarth (1998a, 4) has discussed how research manuals highlight the way in which dress and demeanour may affect the interview interaction, but few have made explicit the impact of the researcher role on the emotional well-being of the researcher. This confusion about the role is made more difficult by the increasing immersion in the social world of the participants that is a hallmark of ethnographic research. For example, one participant came to see me a week after I had conducted an interview and asked whether I did this 'professionally', as his niece was having a problem coming to terms with the death of her mother and he felt it would be really useful for her to talk to me.

On another occasion one participant in the research revealed intensely personal (and distressing) information that was not directly relevant to the research. While this could be considered as verification that trust was established between the interviewee and me, on reflection I realised that I had created (unintentionally) a long pause in the interview, a gap that the interviewee rushed to fill. I realised that the interviewee was probably feeling uncomfortable about the revelation and I felt responsible. The impact of this type of problem on both the researcher and the participants is increased in ethnographic studies as the researcher maintains a presence in the research setting.

Managing the emotional difficulties of conducting research is rarely referred to in the literature with the exception of Howarth (1998a) and Batchelor and Briggs (1994), who argue that support groups and networks amongst those conducting social or medical research could provide a forum in which to share and address the challenges of this work. Clark (2000, 446) has also addressed the issue of the well-being of researchers in palliative care research, suggesting that, just as 'caring for the carers' is part of the ethos of palliative care, there is also a need to support and nurture the researchers.

Ethical considerations

In line with the ethical considerations of informed consent, the right to privacy and protection from harm, a number of procedures were implemented during this research.

Informed consent

Information concerning the research was disseminated in a number of ways. Firstly by letter, with the managers of the various departments in the hospice—chaplaincy, social work, in-patient unit nursing, day care nursing, home care nursing, home care medical and administration. The research included conducting in-depth interviews, and a consent form was presented to each participant prior to commencement, stating the purpose of the research and the voluntary nature of participation. Participants were also alerted to the possibility that the interview might be upsetting and were given information concerning available support mechanisms. The issue of confidentiality was also addressed in the consent form. Although participation in the research was voluntary and it was possible to stop the interview at any time, the existing support mechanisms for staff at the hospice were available, if required.

The right to privacy

I undertook to preserve the anonymity of the participants—by the use of pseudonyms and in some cases by changing the gender of participants and other personal details. The roles of the participants within the organisation, such as nursing or administration staff, have not been changed, as the particular perspective of the participants is an important part of the research. Absolute confidentiality cannot be guaranteed in ethnographic research, however, as already discussed. The small size of the palliative care community in Ireland raises the question of institutional anonymity. This issue was discussed and it was agreed to undertake all reasonable efforts to preserve institutional anonymity. The name and location of the hospice described in the following chapters have been changed, but in spite of this the probability of identification of the hospice remains.

Interviewing terminally ill patients

The research proposal included interviews with terminally ill patients. Permission was received to include day care patients; the nurse manager of the day care would decide the suitability of patients for participation in the research. The criteria used were physical ability to take part, awareness of prognosis and sufficient support systems in place.

During the course of the research and following interviews with nursing staff, permission was extended to include patients from the in-patient unit. Three patients were selected for me to approach about the research. In the case of one potential participant, who was in the hospice for respite care, suitability for participation changed over a weekend. The patient had become distressed at the number of deaths in the four-bedded room. This patient was due for discharge to home, where the support systems—available in the in-patient unit—were not considered adequate if the patient became distressed by the interview.

I spoke to two patients about the research and returned after a few days to see whether they were interested. One patient declined to take part; an interview was conducted with the other patient.

As the research progressed I became uncomfortable about including patients in the research. I increasingly felt that it was inappropriate, although it was not until some months after the research that I could properly explain why I felt this way. A discussion of this aspect of the research and my own sense of unease about including terminally ill patients is presented at the end of Chapter 10, in a section entitled 'Revisiting ethics'. What is clear is that the issue of including terminally ill patients was about the ethical considerations but also part of a reflectiveness that is needed as part and parcel of the research process.

A reflexive process

Boud *et al.* have stated that reflection is an important activity in which people recapture their experience, think about it, mull it over and evaluate it, and working with experience is an important part of learning (1985, 19). In processing experience, Boud *et al.* argue, the way in which this is done is dependent upon the goals and intentions; some of these are clear, as in formal learning tasks, but others are hazy, ill-defined and only become apparent during the research process. Connecting thinking and feelings that are part of the experience with existing attitudes and knowledge can lead to new discoveries (*op. cit.*, 30).

Finlay (2002) strongly advocates that reflexivity be made an explicit aspect of the research process and results, but states that reflexive exploration is 'usually strangled by the constraining word limits set by scientific journals'. Finlay, citing Kvale (1996, 252), describes 'knowledge claims that are so powerful and convincing in their own right that they...carry the validation with them, like a strong piece of art'. Finlay argues that to avoid the reflexive analysis might even compromise the research itself (*op. cit.*, 543). The reflexive process was an ongoing part of this research, although at times hazy and ill-defined, as Boud *et al.* (1985) suggest can be the case, and has been made explicit in the final chapter, in a discussion on interviewing terminally ill patients.

Data analysis

The interviews in this research were recorded and all of the interviews were transcribed. In grounded theory analysis is interwoven with data collection, a process of finding, analysing and theorising. The first few transcripts are interrogated and compared to establish analytical categories that address the research question, are mindful of the research literature and allow the greatest number of data to be coded without forcing or being so numerous as to be meaningless (Glaser and Strauss 1967, 21–3). Glaser and Strauss argue that even if some of the evidence is not entirely accurate this 'will not be too troublesome', for in generating theory 'it is not the fact upon which we stand but the conceptual category' (*op. cit.*, 23). This process involves the researcher in searching for links between categories and searching for emerging themes and theories to see how they stand up to further data. Additional collection of data serves to further facilitate the refinement of initial categories, and the analytical categories are used as sensitising devices that further inform the collection of data.

The opening interview question provided the basis for a number of emergent themes, such as differences between caring and curative health care models, the links between the holistic perspective of palliative care, the values of the organisation and the implications of this for staff. As the research progressed, differences between settings, such as home care or the in-patient unit, began to emerge as health care professionals talked about their own career progression and staff talked about their own experiences as family members. As a result the focus of the later interviews moved toward exploring differences between the care settings and other themes that had emerged from the early interviews.

An initial analysis of the interviews was undertaken as the interview tapes were transcribed. Open coding, i.e. assigning codes to the interview transcripts that made a connection between the research questions and the literature, was conducted with the first fifteen transcripts. These open codes totalled 309, a volume that quickly became unmanageable. These codes were amalgamated into categories, although at this early stage many codes were duplicated within the categories.

A further level of analysis was undertaken at the end of the fieldwork. In line with the conceptual framework, I found it helpful to consider a series of 'maps' (organisation, family, professional roles and so on) and organised the categories within these 'maps'. Considering these themes or categories in this way helped me to visualise how they might fit together or overlap. This conceptualisation started a process of thinking about the relationships (between patients and family members, patients and professional staff, and professional staff and families) and how they may be shaped and influenced by the location of care.

Kellehear (1998) has discussed qualitative research analysis, which, he argues, can become overwhelmed by anxieties or methods that more truly belong to quantitative research. He uses as an example the increasing tendency in qualitative research to use qualitative analysis software and makes an amusing response to queries regarding aids that he uses for analysis:

> *'I sing the praises of a HB pencil. I am also partial to red pens. I have found these technologies quite complementary to the "software" between my ears—my own imagination, thinking ability and perceptions (a software package known as BRAIN)'* (1998, 16).

Kellehear makes a valid point; while qualitative analysis software does have a use, I found it best merely to use it as a tool for electronic indexing and sorting of material. This research used NVivo software to 'code up' from written notes and coding originally made on transcripts. Moving segments of texts around and ordering the text within categories was certainly made less tedious by using this software. There is, however, no shortcut to the long reflective process involved in digesting, mulling over and endlessly considering the huge amount of information that has been collected. The moments of inspiration often happened when not focusing on the material—often in the shower or when out walking—when a vague thought on the horizon of my mind suddenly came into sharper focus and a thread of connection was made. The NVivo software, and other similar packages, certainly aided the physical working out of that connection but they did not, and cannot, make the connection.

Summary

The aim of this study was to explore how a 'good death' and the spiritual dimension of care were understood from a variety of perspectives within a palliative care setting in Ireland and to further explore whether there was a cultural specificity to these concepts. The research was an ethnographic study using a grounded theory approach. The difficulty of attaining absolute confidentiality in ethnographic research was addressed, as were the ethical considerations of the research, in particular those concerning interviewing terminally ill patients; this issue will be revisited in Chapter 10.

The research used observation and in-depth interviews as a means of gathering information. Forty-seven interviews were conducted with a variety of staff in the hospice. Names and in some cases gender have been changed in the extracts presented in the following chapters, although the occupation of the participants has been retained.

SECTION 2
A VIEW OF PALLIATIVE CARE IN IRELAND

INTRODUCTION

This section presents five chapters that can be considered as a series of 'sketch-maps' portraying, with increasing focus, a view of palliative care culture in Ireland. These chapters are largely descriptive and set out the social landscape. In cartographic terms, they are similar to the landscape sketches of early explorers and depict with broad brush strokes the culture of palliative care. The way in which the key aspects of palliative care—communication and open awareness, and the concept of 'total pain' and the means of uncovering multi-dimensional pain through multi-disciplinary working—are enacted within palliative care in Ireland is described. The relationships between individuals, family members and professional staff and the organisation are described and considered in terms of location of care. Chapters 7 and 8 describe differences between religion and spirituality and how a 'good death' is understood. The section begins with a brief description of the hospice where the research was conducted (the names of the organisation and staff have been changed). The values of the Catholic religious order who established the hospice have shaped the organisation that runs this palliative care service. The aims of palliative care, outlined in Section 1, are interwoven with those of the organisation, and the impact of this is considered.

The research setting

Many hospices in the UK and Ireland were established by voluntary groups, as discussed in Chapters 1 and 2. In Ireland hospices were also established by Catholic religious orders, with much of the infrastructure such as land and buildings being provided by the orders. Some hospices are located in their original buildings and additional new buildings, in some cases, have been constructed on land belonging to the religious orders.

Palliative care was spearheaded by the Sisters of Charity at Our Lady's Hospice in Dublin, and while these religious sisters have been instrumental in providing services, other religious orders and voluntary groups have followed their example and developed services around the country. Many of these services are now funded by the Department of Health and Children although fund-raising remains an important source of income for all palliative care services.

The best of everything

The research was conducted at St Theresa's Hospice, established by the Sisters of Mary, a Catholic order of nuns involved in health care in Ireland. I had the opportunity to talk with one of the founders of the hospice, Sr Bridget, who explained that the original aim was to establish a home care service, but the current hospice had quickly developed as the need for the service grew and the public support for the hospice, by way of fund-raising, was substantial. This public support facilitated the rapid expansion of the service and new buildings for the hospice.

Sr Bridget's own philosophy of 'having the best of everything' was evident in the design and structures of the new buildings and in the interior decoration of the hospice, which featured high-quality furniture and furnishings. Although the religious sisters were the principal organisers and providers of initial funding for the services, religious pictures and artefacts such as crucifixes were kept to a minimum and could be easily removed. Sheila, one of the doctors at the hospice, explained that 'thought had gone into what should be displayed', for instance in the number of religious icons on display. Her own view, however, was that the hospice was a Catholic institution and the involvement of the religious order was a very positive involvement that also needed to be acknowledged.

> *'There is thought gone into this, there are all the religious icons for instance but none of them are fixed to the walls, you know, you can just lift it off. So if somebody comes in, if we are admitting a Muslim for whom a crucifix is offensive you can just take it off.... it is not completely part of the structure, but it is there. I wouldn't like to see any more religious pictures and we get donations of holy pictures, none of which are ever put up.... We also have to respect the religious order who are involved here and their involvement is part of what makes the place as good as it is.'* (Sheila, doctor, par. 231)

St Theresa's Hospice

St Theresa's Hospice provided a range of services—in-patient services, day care and home care—and buildings had been added over the years as the service expanded. In the main building a corridor led from the reception area to the in-patient unit and to the lower floor, where the canteen, the laundry rooms and the mortuary were situated. At the end of this corridor from the reception area, a small chapel faced back toward the reception area. To one side of the chapel there were two single rooms which were used for more independent patients, and to the left of the chapel the in-patient unit began. The two single rooms were not immediately apparent to the eye, as they were tucked away into an alcove to the right of the chapel and seemed isolated and set apart from the main in-patient unit. The chapel, on the other hand, was dominant and, although a pleasing and restful space, it felt like a gateway to the in-patient unit.

The chapel was not an overtly Catholic setting, although it was clearly a religious and reflective space, with soft light from a large stained-glass window; there was a small central altar with fifteen or so chairs on either side. The room was often filled with flowers. Religious and generally reflective books and pamphlets were placed on a small shelf on one of the sidewalls of the chapel. Many people, staff and family members and perhaps patients—although I never saw any there except during Mass—seemed to pop in and out during the day and evening and sit quietly.

Offices for the ward manager and the medical staff were located close to the in-patient unit. Many of the administration staff also had offices here and this was where I was allocated office space. The canteen was situated close to the in-patient unit and going through the in-patient unit was a quicker route to the canteen; however, staff were encouraged to take a longer and more circuitous route in order to maintain a quiet atmosphere and protect patient privacy.

A Catholic place

Although some members of staff expressed a view that thought had been given to presenting a non-religious, or at least a minimally religious, environment, it was obvious, certainly to me, that St Theresa's was associated with a religious, and Catholic, order. Sheila, although reared as a Catholic but no longer practising, was concerned about the impression people may have of the hospice, and although she noticed some aspects, such as Catholic newspapers and magazines around the place, she felt that she was still not sufficiently distant from the culture of Catholicism to notice quite how the hospice may appear to non-Catholics.

> *'This is a Catholic institute and one of the problems is if you grow up in a Catholic environment you may not notice how Catholic some places are. I came in here one Monday morning and there are copies of the* Irish Catholic *all over the place and I gathered them up. The* Irish Catholic *is quite a conservative paper and if you walk in and every table has a copy of the* Irish Catholic, *it gives a different impression. So I think it is okay to have a copy of the* Irish Catholic, *that's fine, but not to walk down the main corridor and the* Irish Catholic *is the only thing that is lying about. Very often the magazines are donated and the good ones get nicked. And the ones that don't get nicked are the magazines like the* Sacred Heart. Hello *magazine might land on the table and is gone again, the magazines from the missionary societies tend to be nice easy reads with pictures. And they are grand but nobody wants to steal them. I was brought up in a Catholic environment but I am not a Catholic. But I still find I am not distant enough to be able to see how Catholic this place looks to a non-Catholic.'* (Sheila, doctor)

For many of the staff, however, the presence of a Catholic religious order at the hospice and the Christian ethos that underpinned the care of staff, patients and family members was a very positive aspect. Jean, who worked in administration at St Theresa's, welcomed the availability of daily religious services and the opportunity for occasional religious reflections.

> *'I was delighted when I came here and there was the Easter reflection. If you want to go to Mass on a Holy Day it's there. You know, it's convenient for me and not everybody would use the facilities and that's up to them. You see they are set up in place, there is complete tolerance of everybody, like everybody is different, it doesn't matter what your circumstances are, you know whether you are married, divorced, single parent, whatever. Every-*

> *body is just the same from that point of view. So that is good, it's not that we are a very religious place here.'* (Jean, administration)

Although the organisation is a Catholic one, Elizabeth felt that it was the Christian ethos of care, rather than a specifically Catholic view, that informed the organisational values at St Theresa's.

> *'There is nothing like, like there aren't crucifixes hanging, you know, there is nothing like that. There is just a sense that Christian care is at the heart of it all.'* (Elizabeth, administration)

CHAPTER 4

The experience of palliative care

Introduction

The influence of the ethos and the organisational values seemed to complement and enhance the practice of palliative care at St Theresa's. The nature of the model of palliative care, its aims and practices, and the contrasting experience of health care in other settings influenced and shaped the perceptions of patients, families and professionals.

Curative and care models

Palliative care aims to care for patients and families holistically when cure is no longer possible, as discussed in Chapter 1, and this is in contrast to general health care, which is based on a curative model, addresses a diverse range of illnesses and, as its name suggests, focuses on cure. The contrasting experiences of health care within the two models of care have influenced and shaped the perceptions of the care in the hospice by family members and staff.

I found that family members and professional staff painted a bleak picture of the care available in general hospitals. The type of personal treatment given and received had a big impact on patients and family members; this was often a negative experience within general hospitals and a very positive one in palliative care services, which tended to shape the perceptions of the care in the hospice. In a hospital setting, staff experienced difficulties with the lack of time and resources to care for patients because of the restraints of the task-focused curative model and staff shortages. Many of the nursing staff were frustrated by the organisational structures, resources and values of the organisation which did not facilitate the caring aspect of the nursing role. In contrast, the palliative care model not only facilitated this aspect but emphasised it, and for staff and family members this made a huge difference.

Contrasting experiences

The focus on individual needs and on family members in palliative care services seemed to transform the impact of the illness and death for family members and the patient. Elizabeth, in her job at reception in St Theresa's, had a lot of contact with family members and was aware of the positive impact of the hospice on families and patients.

> *'Then for other people, some people come in from hospital and they cannot get over the way they are treated here because it is so different. It's so kind.'* (Elizabeth, administration)

The views of family members

The positive comments made by family members about the hospice highlighted how difficult the hospital experience was for some families. Helen, whose husband had died at the hospice and who now worked there, expressed how she thought families felt when they come from hospital to hospice care. Even the small detail of addressing patients and family members by their name left a huge impression.

> *'This is why so many families, you know, they just cannot believe the difference, you know. To be addressed by your first name, they are interested, they want to know how you are. It's just that sense of caring and that you are important.'* (Helen, family member and administration)

Although patients may have had years of hospital treatment and only a short time at the hospice, the impact of this contrast was considerable. Sally, a home care nurse who trained in palliative care nursing after her father spent his last ten days in the care of a hospice, felt that even those few days transformed the experience for herself and her father.

> *'We went to different hospitals and between them all, he got no dignity... he got ten days in the hospice and those ten days changed his life and mine. Because whatever they did and it didn't cost money, they gave him back his dignity.'* (Sally, home care nurse)

Helen was overwhelmed by the consideration shown to her and her family, and this was a big contrast with her long and difficult time in the hospital system.

> *'I have very much seen it from both sides of the fence. I was so overwhelmed by the kindness and the care and the support that just wasn't there for so many years in dealing with the hospital system, which I had with Tom [her husband]. He had a long haul and ... there was constant hospital contacts which at the best of time you felt you were a file and number. It was very very difficult, the lack of communication and fighting, fighting for his needs. It just became a constant struggle and I absolutely believe, I will never be able to express how much the difference in just the care, immediately embraced and not just the patient, it was the whole family, and they very quickly got to know me. And it was your needs and they very much take their lead from you.'*(Helen, family member and administration)

Continuance of care for the family after the death is part of the service at St Theresa's, and this again was a huge contrast to the often-abrupt end to the contact with the hospital once the patient died. Jean talked about the experience of her father's sudden death in hospital ten years ago. Her only contact with the hospital afterwards was to collect his death certificate.

> *'When people come into the hospice you can say you are going to have follow-up as well but again in my time in the hospital there was nothing and I think that was the hard part. You know, "Your father's dead, go home now." What happened after that, no follow-up, nothing, I just went to get the death cert. and that's your last... It's such a contrast, here is such a contrast to my experience of death, people are lucky to be able to avail of these services, as hard as it is at least you have the follow-up.'* (Jean, administration)

The views of professional staff

Family members talked about the care at the hospice in very warm terms and clearly felt supported. Their appreciation of the kindness and attention of the staff suggested that their previous experience in the hospital system was very poor. The type of care and support that the hospice provided was facilitated in a number of ways—by the aims of the model of care, the organisational values and by the actions of the staff, all of which are connected.

Firstly, the purpose and outcome of the palliative care model is clear; there is the inevitability of the death of the patient in a hospice, whereas the remit and focus of hospital settings is on cure. Death within a curative model is a failure; within palliative care, the focus is on how good that death can be. For the nursing staff, for whom caring is an inherent part of their work role, the palliative care model provided the opportunity to develop and focus on that aspect of their work, a focus that may not be so easily incorporated within the task focus of the curative model. Three of the nurses, Emer, Christine and Marie, spoke about the setting and the focus, and the difference these aspects made. Although people do die in hospital, the aims of the hospital are to diagnose, treat and cure people, and hospital, in their view, was not a suitable place for people to die.

> *'An emergency room in a hospital is not a place for people to die. The mandate of a hospital is diagnose, treat and cure. The mandate is not to have people die.'* (Emer, nurse)

Christine also emphasised that, in contrast to the hospital setting, every patient who came into the hospice was going to die. Christine also talked about the difficulties of being unable to give dying patients, in a hospital setting, the kind of care she felt they needed.

> *'It is a very different environment, totally different. I think why it is so different, is that everyone who comes in is ultimately going to die—compared to an active setting in a general hospital where a number of people will die and you will struggle with that because you are not able to give them the level of care that you might like to.'* (Christine, nurse)

The aims of the two models are different and consequently there are different values associated with each. The shift from a task focus to a patient focus in the hospice reflected a different value system, one that is quite the reverse of a hospital.

> *'If you think of a general hospital your value system is, six patients in the morning getting them up, getting them dressed and looking nice and if you do that you are a good nurse. Here your value system is what have you dealt with today and what have you done, she said, like, she was dying and I said this and, like, it is valued... the spiritual care is valued as well, but in the hospitals it is not.'* (Marie, nurse)

The hospice seemed to accommodate patient needs in ways that would not be possible in a general and larger health care setting.

> *'In a general hospital or acute hospital you will try to facilitate somebody if they don't want their breakfast now but it is a nuisance, but here it is not a nuisance, you know, you try to do at the patient's pace, at whatever they wish.'* (Bernadette, chaplain)

> *'Anything goes when it come to patients, if a patient wants fillet steak, they will get into the car and go and get it, that is a must.'* (Carmel, kitchen staff)

The emphasis on task rather than care within the curative model frustrated some of the nursing staff in this study. Christine felt that it contrasted with her personal perception and understanding of the nature of care. While the curative model also incorporates care, an unintended consequence of this model may be an overemphasis on tasks rather than a balance between care and tasks. Caring for people holistically seemed to correspond more closely with an understanding of the nature of care, particularly from a nursing perspective, and for many of the staff that I spoke with this seemed to be a major attraction for working within palliative care.

> *'Within a hospital setting, from my experience and it was something that eventually drove me into hospice because I struggled with knowing that what the patient actually needed was more of a total holistic approach. But there was the time constraint and the personnel restraint so you had to focus on getting tasks done... I would not have satisfaction from my job unless I could link in with somebody on a more human level. However, [in hospital] I would have found myself at times, not asking an open-ended question because I didn't have the time to listen.'* (Christine, nurse)

The influence of organisational structures and values

The practice of the palliative care model seemed to be enhanced by the organisational structures and values at St Theresa's. This was apparent in a number of ways and a strong theme to emerge in the research was the importance of equity of service. This policy, which operates in St Theresa's, contrasts with the general health service in Ireland and some other palliative care services in Ireland. The commitment to high levels of nursing staff to meet patient needs was also considered an important feature of the care in the hospice.

Sr Bridget's view that 'small is beautiful' seemed to carry through to various aspects of the hospice, such as the scale and size of the original buildings, familiarity between staff and family members, and the attention to small details in the care of patients. A further aspect of the organisational values was an appreciation of the commitment and contribution of all the staff, and an attention to their needs as well as those of patients and family members. The provision of a caring and supportive environment for staff seemed to increase the existing staff commitment to the work and the organisation.

Equity of service

St Theresa's operated an admission policy to the in-patient unit which was assessed on a needs basis and there were no costs to the patient or the family for any aspect of the service provided, including home care or day care. This contrasts with the two-tiered health service that operates in general health care in Ireland and other palliative care services.

The impetus for this emphasis on and commitment to equity of service seemed to originate with Sr Bridget and the philosophy of care of the Sisters of Mary, a commitment that continued with the management team at the hospice. Sr Bridget told me a story about the first referrals the hospice received. On the first day of the service in 1989, two women were referred, both of whom were called Helen. One Helen was a professional lady who lived in an affluent suburb close to the hospice; the other Helen came from a deprived area closer to the city. Sr Bridget derived great pleasure from knowing that both these women received the same treatment and at no cost to themselves, and for her they came to represent a symbol of the quality and equity of the service.

Equity of service was a theme that wove its way through many of the interviews and was an important aspect for staff, as well as for patients and family members. One new member of staff was attracted to a post in the hospice because of it, and commented in the hospice newsletter that it 'spoke volumes about the ethos of the place'.

Jean had contact with families about the availability of beds in the hospice and explained the categorisation system for assessing patient need. An example of this are home care patients, who were considered in greater need than patients already in the hospital system as these patients had nursing care; when this was explained to families on the waiting list, this transparency seemed to be welcomed and appreciated.

> *'If you have somebody in a hospital bed, they are getting nursing, getting medical input, whereas if there is somebody at home with family trying to cope, they will always come in ahead of a hospital patient. It's very fair, it's great that you can be so open with people and say that to people and I am quite comfortable in saying that to families and they always understand.'* (Jean, administration)

Jean also enjoyed the equity and fairness of the system, especially when it meant that people who had hard lives had some comfort at the end of their lives.

> *'Everybody is equal, to see people who may have been homeless or people who have nobody, we get a lot of people who maybe have had hard lives on their own and to see them come in and at least have the comfort of here. It's so brilliant, it's such a fair system and I can really stand over it because I am involved in it, it's really the person who needs to come next will come and it doesn't matter who you are.'* (Jean, administration)

A clear admissions policy, not influenced by personal contacts, was another aspect of this transparency that was important to staff.

> *'I remember there was somebody from the government who was a friend of this person on the waiting list. They were on the phone about six times. I said this to the doctor, "They have been on the phone again", and she looked at me and said "That cuts no ice with me, it's how ill they are". I was real impressed, that's the way it should be.'* (Susan, administration)

Within the hospice, the allocation of the resources was also on a needs basis. For instance, patients were allocated single rooms in the in-patient unit, if they were available, on a needs basis rather than single rooms being considered as private health care facilities, which was the case in hospitals and some other hospices.

> *'The level of care in the single rooms would be appropriate for the level of care needed rather than nursing as a private room.'* (Karen, nurse)

Need was assessed on a number of different levels. Susan told me that in several cases the single room was allocated to a parent with young children, who was seen as having a greater need to spend time with his or her family than some of the other patients.

> *'It doesn't matter who you are or what level of cover, that doesn't come into it. It's, like, just people with young families; there is man there with young children, moved down the other day to a single room because he has young children. And just privacy, so his wife and children can come in and that's why they moved him.'* (Susan, administration)

Although the equity of service demonstrated at St Theresa's was important to staff and patients and laudable in the context of health care services in Ireland, St Theresa's provided an equitable service for cancer patients only. The ethical issues concerning the allocation of these resources to limited patient groups are pertinent and have already been discussed in Chapter 1.

Size of organisation and service

The original vision for St Theresa's was of a small-scale home care service. The level of referrals to the service drove an expansion that was not originally anticipated. Concerns were expressed by some of the medical and nursing staff that the developmental changes, although largely welcomed, would displace the intimate atmosphere in the hospice. Staff who had been working at St Theresa's for a long time were particularly concerned and worried that the development might erode the personal approach by staff to the care of the patients and family members. This personal approach was perceived by staff to be present even in the details of the physical environment, such as the absence of institutional-type signs outside and inside the physical building. Just as consideration was given to the number and type of religious pictures on the interior walls, a similar view was taken of not providing signs in order to enhance a homely and intimate atmosphere.

> *'There are no signs, so people have to ask their way.'* (Elizabeth, administration)

The smallness of the in-patient building and the physical location of the reception area, as a central entrance point into the building, necessitated meeting reception staff and was, according to Marie, one of the nurses at St Theresa's, a positive benefit and promoted a familiarity with staff that she felt was only possible in a small organisation.

> *'The smallness of it too, you get a nice atmosphere, you know the receptionist here when you walk in here... when you are greeted by somebody you automatically warm to the place whereas if you are greeted by "go down the corridor and turn right", you know it is such a difference.'* (Marie, nurse)

The home care team, which became two teams by the end of my research, was small in size and this, according to Marie, helped the development of relationships with patients and family.

> *'You see, in the smaller team you know them a lot more, you have got a sense of them from listening to them, but when you have got a big team you don't visit the same few people at the same time because you are covering a bigger range or area.'* (Marie, nurse)

In the in-patient unit, Sally, a nurse who had also experienced palliative care as a family member, felt that the emphasis on the person and the small personal touches made a profound difference to the patient and the family.

> *'The nice little things like a cloth under their water glass, you know, just nice things, it was so simple. And I am not talking about the symptom control. It was what I perceived as a relative because there was good symptom control, but there were all those other things that did make the difference... it was just, it was nothing big, it was just the way they greeted you.'* (Sally, nurse and family member)

Staff–patient ratio

The focus on responding to patient and family need rather than on accomplishing tasks demands a large number of nursing and care staff.

> *'I think hospice lends itself to that, you are better staffed than in a general setting. The whole approach is if this person needs me for an hour, there is an understanding on the team that you can allow somebody to be with somebody for as long as that person needs them. Provided you have told your colleagues "I am going in to room six or whatever and I don't know how long I am going to be" the patients get the time they need, as far as possible we do try to give them as much time as they need.'* (Christine, nurse)

Margaret, one of the medical staff, felt that the palliative care services had a protection from cutbacks of staff that other areas of health care did not.

> *'The one thing that palliative care has that other areas don't is protection of high staff to patient ratios.'* (Margaret, doctor)

Although there was a high staff to patient ratio, the clinical aspect was very small compared to other settings, but staff felt they were as busy as professionals in acute or general health care settings.

> *'We have much higher levels here than would be in any ward in any hospital*

> *and even with that we would be rushed off our feet. But our rushed off our feet would be different from a hospital. Our rushed off our feet might be from talking to a patient for an hour to sitting down talking to the family for half an hour to doing our rounds and sitting down and talking to someone else. The clinical element of the care is tiny compared to everything else.'* (Geraldine, nurse)

Working in harmony

The professional staff work within a shared philosophy of care, and this approach engendered a sense of working toward a common aim in harmony with other staff members and being supported, organisationally, to do so.

> *'We're very privileged and we have the luxury in this service of people thinking along the same lines, the same approach to family, friends, relevant others. You don't have the conflicts that you have in hospitals, so it's easier to work in. You are all sort of going the same way and you are well supported. There is an awareness of what we are all about, what we are doing and you are not going in different directions. And it is a great luxury to have, you know, time and staffing and support.'* (Catherine, nurse)

Bernadette, one of the chaplains for the in-patient unit in St Theresa's, had previously worked as a nurse in an acute hospital and felt that people 'thought differently' in the hospice and consequently there was a more peaceful atmosphere.

> *'I don't think it could be compared to an acute hospital, I honestly feel that having worked here for six months that it is a totally different set up, everybody is thinking differently and there is that sense of peace and just moving along.'* (Bernadette, chaplain)

Organisational values

Throughout the time I spent at St Theresa's I felt very welcome and that my research work was valued. Sr Aileen, one of the senior management team, often stopped me in the corridor to ask me how things were going, and Sr Maura, another senior staff member, who loved the focus on spiritual care that was part of my research, always grabbed my arm firmly every time we met to tell me I was doing 'great work'. I really liked the positive appreciation of the research, and as a consequence I could see myself becoming very committed to St Theresa's. This commitment was a feeling that many staff seemed to share.

> *'I think it's great to say that you work somewhere and you would be happy to be here as a patient or be happy to have anybody in and it's great to be able to say that. And it's great for me to be able to say that to families, "I can assure you that you will get the best care, or your family will have the best care." It's great to believe in something so much.'* (Jean, administration).

The focus of care, at St Theresa's and in palliative care generally, is on the patient and the family. At St Theresa's this focus on the person also seemed to be reflected in dealings with members of staff; for instance, family difficulties experienced by staff seemed to be met with understanding and support. Geraldine, a nurse in the hospice, had family problems which had led her to be absent for a while, and she was overwhelmed by the support she had received from her nursing manager and her colleagues.

> *'My experience is that I couldn't have got any more support than I got here. I got so much support from the highest right down. Everyone across the board have been absolutely fantastic and I know I wouldn't be here now only for them.'* (Geraldine, nurse)

Marie, another nurse, had a similar experience.

> *'I know once ringing in sick and I was having problems at home and it was "Of course your family come first", straight away, of course your family come first, you know, take a week off, that to me just said an awful lot.'* (Marie, nurse)

The organisational focus and support and an acknowledgement of commitment by staff seemed to be reciprocated by staff, and resulted in an increase in staff commitment.

'If you are treated well you give more and you are valued, like, if you are just one of a number in a hospital you don't give. If what you do does not make a difference why bother, but if you do here then they say you did awful well, when you come back you can feel you have done well.' (Marie, nurse)

The size of the organisation and the presence of the religious sisters gave a feeling of the organisation as a family and of the hospice as a home; these aspects seemed to reinforce a feeling of intimacy and familiarity.

'I don't know if it is the sisters or whatever it is but it is a more homely place. It is small; they value you whereas if you have people that are part of the health board it is just a job. It is more homely, if you are coming from a base where you feel valued, you know, you go off out there with much more and you give much more whereas if you are one of a number you are just going to do the job.' (Marie, nurse)

The values and culture of the organisation fostered and supported the commitment of staff. Jean felt that this was to do with the presence of the religious sisters. In her experience, this was a benefit as there was always 'extra things' such as consideration for the spiritual needs of staff. She also felt, however, that the clergy and the religious sisters, because of their vocation and singular focus, were able to give a huge commitment to their work, a commitment they expected from staff, in spite of other obligations staff may have.

'We have these extra things and probably if we had no sisters we wouldn't have that. So the spiritual needs of staff are looked after from that point of view as well. But the sisters can be difficult as well in their own way. They are doing their job and this is... not all they have to do, but this is their focus and they can give 120%. But you have another life which you have to go home to and start when you leave. It's their vocation, it's not your vocation. I think that they can be demanding, the clergy overall, the sisters and the priests because they expect, and I do myself, I give 100% to my job and I expect everyone else to do the same. We all do but I suppose they give 100% vocation and they expect maybe a little bit of that. So sometimes that

can be a disadvantage, but I think the advantages outweigh it.' (Jean, administration)

A supportive environment

One of the aims of palliative care is to provide support for patients and their families. At St Theresa's this support was present on a number of different levels, from maintaining a professional relationship with the patient when other health professionals have nothing more to offer, to providing a safe and supportive physical environment. This type of care and support, however, placed considerable demands on the professional and other staff, who in turn need to be supported in their work.

Supporting patients and family members

The hospice aimed to provide a supportive environment for patients who were often perceived to be isolated, vulnerable and abandoned by a health care system that could do nothing further to help them in their illness.

> *'They are getting support. That is a big thing that we provide for them. Probably the most negative things that can be said to a patient and they say it sometimes in a general hospital is at the end. The doctor will say "There is nothing more I can offer you"...and then people's concerns are "I have been very unwell, I am now dying and you are telling me it's bye-bye and I am off home to die on my own".'* (Margaret, doctor)

Within the hospice, the singular focus of care and on death and dying provided an opportunity to explore the reality of terminal illness in what was perceived by staff to be a supportive physical environment.

> *'Another thing that people would comment on about here... it is so calm here so I think we provide an atmosphere to allow people to work through their thoughts and to face, to help them face what is ahead. Very hard in a ward when there are trolleys coming in and out and some guy is going to surgery and having something else and somebody else is having something.'* (Margaret, doctor)

Supporting staff

The provision of palliative care with the inherent engagement at a personal level with the patient and family members was personally rewarding and satisfying for many of the staff; however, it was also personally demanding. In supporting patients and their families, the staff I spoke to in this research identified the need for adequate support structures to be in place, organisationally and professionally. Nevertheless, staff also identified that, in meaningfully engaging with patients, a degree of self-awareness concerning the demands on themselves was required. This awareness required practitioners to put in place some mechanism of self-support.

> *'I have my own coping mechanism well in place; unless I am able to assess the situations and see whether I am getting stressed and what is causing that stress. If there is the build-up of grief or build-up of trauma then I really need to address that at an individual level.'* (Christine, nurse)

The need for staff support was recognised at management level, and although Sheila felt that it was important for the organisation to facilitate and provide support, some balance was needed in order to find the appropriate level of support.

> *'You don't want a kind of macho culture that if you want any support at all you are a complete wimp but at the same time you don't want a culture, an organisation that its function is to provide staff support rather than to provide care, so there is that kind of balancing.'* (Sheila, doctor)

There was a recognition that providing this type of care for patients placed demands on individuals and those who work in the organisation at different areas and levels.

> *'If we want to maintain what we have now we need to focus on individuals, carers, and I mean from the kitchen staff to the social workers to the volunteers. Everyone brings their own aspect of care. If we want to maintain the quality of care that we are giving then we need to be careful that we don't stretch people beyond their limits.'* (Christine, nurse)

While formal support was available, much of the support came from colleagues in a less formal way. For some staff, particularly home care team members who work in isolation much of the time, returning to the hospice and meeting with colleagues seemed to provide this level of support.

> *'I think a lot of it is to do with the team structure because you are very well supported within the team. When you come back, you can talk to somebody about it. You can talk to your colleagues, you have a very good social worker that you can go and look to for guidance and you can say, I am stuck here, I don't know where I am going, I don't know what I am doing. We have a meeting once a week and talk about issues. If you are stuck with something you know that you can offload as well and you can get a new focus on that or what to do with it. Or if it is just too much you can say look it is just too much, you need a break, let somebody else go in there with another new perspective.'* (Marie, nurse)

Sometimes the level of support was nothing more than having the opportunity to tell the story of what has happened.

Currently palliative care services in Ireland are not at the same developmental stage, and while professional expertise is at a similar level, the levels of services available, in terms of numbers of hospices and home care teams, are considerably less and the health care system is different.

> *'The differences in the UK would be they would probably have a better country cover than we do but that is expanding now, there are now hospices in different regions and new consultants being appointed all the time. I don't know, maybe the UK is better developed in dealing with different ethnic groups than we are and that is something we have only had to begin to deal with in the last year.'* (Margaret, doctor)

In this study, palliative care professionals who had experienced working within the UK system commented on the organisational focus on symptom management rather than a focus on holistic care that included comprehensive psychosocial and spiritual care.

> *'You couldn't say the UK as a big block. I worked in one hospice, there was*

> *a very strong move there to symptom management, and there was a very strong lip service to comprehensive care... If the accepted norm is that a specialist palliative care unit has an average stay of eight days and a nursing home for the dying has an average stay of twenty-one days, you don't want to be a nursing home for the dying, you want to be a hospice. Therefore, you drive to have a short length of stay. You try to have a short length of stay by admitting people with uncomplicated problems or by only dealing with what you can deal with. They are only dealing with the physical side of things. Therefore you don't admit people with complicated psychosocial problems, you either say that is not your remit or that all pre-dates that cancer or, you know you say a whole range of things.'* (Sheila, doctor)

Cultural differences

There were also other perceived differences between palliative care in the UK and Ireland that reflect a particular cultural emphasis and modes of interaction. These mainly concern the overall influence of the Catholic Church within health care.

Catholic organisation

Historically, the presence of religious orders within the health service and their traditional involvement in nurse training, discussed in Chapter 2, has made the inclusion of religious ceremonies and rituals within health care settings a normal practice. While there was a religious order directly involved in St Theresa's, this is also the case in many other hospices in Ireland, although some hospices and regional home care services are managed and funded by regional health board authorities. As already discussed in Chapter 2, the majority of the population in Ireland is Catholic, and the majority of palliative care patients are Catholic and elderly. The presence of religious, nuns and priests and the availability of daily Mass and other religious sacraments seemed to be important for many patients and some members of staff.

> *'Ireland still has high church attendance, particularly in the age group we are dealing with. The actual formal liturgical spirituality stuff, that is an important part, you know, seeing priests, nuns, prayer, that's very important*

> *for people. And I think that is something that is done well here at the hospice.'* (Sheila, doctor)

Although the Irish population is predominantly Catholic, it was clear from talking to people in this study that not everyone embraced Catholicism to the same degree. Given the recent revelations of physical and sexual abuse in Catholic institutions, discussed in Chapter 2, it was clear that many people had difficult and painful experiences with the Catholic Church. While the impact of these difficulties is discussed in a later chapter, one difficulty is a lack of choice concerning hospice beds, as these are mainly provided by Catholic religious orders.

In St Theresa's the religious order tried very hard to be inclusive but the Catholic nature of the organisation was still evident, as discussed earlier. While consideration was given to the visible signs of a Catholic presence, there was Mass almost every day in the chapel, attended mostly by day care patients, and the chaplain visited each room in the in-patient unit, unless expressly requested not to, with Holy Communion every day. This level of Catholic and religious activity was not part of the home care service, although a chaplain was available to call on home visits.

The lack of choice of services elsewhere may lead patients to conform to the dominant culture of the organisation when admitted to the hospice for respite or terminal care. Margaret, one of the hospice doctors, tried to explain how patients might have felt on coming into the hospice, if they were not particularly religious.

> *'The only thing on a patient's mind might be that hospice care in the area is run by a religious order and they can talk all they like about spiritual but that's Catholic. And this is a Catholic who you know burnt his bridges with God twenty years ago so everybody in there is Catholic and if he goes in there, he is thinking I'll shut my mouth.'* (Margaret, doctor)

Owing to the involvement of Catholic organisations in many of the state institutions as discussed in Chapter 2, politeness, which many people referred to, may be a learned response in a predominantly Catholic culture.

> *'Some people can be too polite, now there has been one or two who would say "I would prefer if you didn't come" but that would be very few.'* (Bernadette, chaplain)

Although Ireland is predominantly Catholic, how this Catholicism is practised has changed. There can be an assumption, not restricted to the hospice, that most elderly people are religious and Catholic, although some of the staff, particularly those who had worked in other countries, seemed aware of making assumptions about religious beliefs and practices.

> *'We were talking about spiritual care. There were some nurses there and one of them said to me "In our hospital they put the rosary over the loudspeaker every day", it wasn't a hospital, it was a nursing home. Now that is an assumption that everybody likes to say the rosary every day. I said to her "Why would you do that"? And she said "Well, they are older people and they probably like it", but I said "One day I am going to be old and do not do that with me".'* (Emer, nurse)

Religious focus

The religious, and predominantly Catholic, presence in health care services has led to a development of and emphasis on the psychosocial and spiritual aspects of care that extends beyond the perimeters of pastoral or nursing care, as demonstrated by the work of Michael Kearney and discussed in Chapter 2.

> *'I found this area was highly developed in Ireland, it is one of the areas that it is known elsewhere for… there are people who have been over here and are impressed and Michael Kearney in Harold's Cross is writing a lot and is well known.'* (Joan, social worker)

The presence of a religious ethos was also the norm in other social institutions such as education, and this presence may portray what seemed to be a 'naturalness' of religion within Irish culture.

> *'In England, they were more multi-cultural but for a lot from a Christian or*

> *Catholic background, there was a lot of non-practising Catholics. So you might have just the ritual of attending to the prayers just before the person died, or actually as the person died. Whereas in Ireland, now this is a generalisation as there are a lot of changes here, more lapsed people and that, but overall, particularly for the older generation, religion was more of an integrated part of their journey. And I suppose that is the difference, in Ireland you are living in a very religious background really...You are living in a culture where religion is a very natural thing, because religion is very much a natural part of Irish culture.'* (Christine, nurse)

Not all the professional staff, however, especially those who have worked outside Ireland, considered the 'naturalness' of a religious ethos a positive feature. Catherine talked about her experience of palliative care nursing overseas, where there was no set religious practice for dying people, and how she noticed the pervasiveness of religious practices in Ireland, although there was not a very overtly Catholic environment.

> *'The sky didn't fall in because the candles weren't lit and because there was another way of doing things that I hadn't been aware of. So when I came back here to work I found it very overpowering in terms of the religious impact. Although there's not, looking around there's not sort of statues everywhere and you know it's very low key but still the whole, there is the Irish attitude to death —get the candles, you know, it's time to light the candles, you know they're about to die—I found that very strange.'* (Catherine, nurse)

Summary

This chapter has considered the research setting of St Theresa's Hospice. The traditional involvement of religious orders in health care and other social institutions in Ireland has led to a sense of 'naturalness' about the presence of religious orders and religious practice in these settings. It would seem from the views of participants in the study that the religious order which established and was involved in running the hospice also influenced the organisational values, which in turn seemed to enhance the delivery of palliative care and provided a supportive environment for staff, patients and families. The level of support for staff working in the hospice seemed to have an expansive rather than contracting effect on the level of commitment and belief in the organisation, in contrast to commitment and belief in the general health service.

The perception of palliative care by patients, families and staff was a very positive one; however, this perception appeared to be greatly influenced by the contrasting and often quite negative experience of the health service in Ireland. Staff, particularly nursing staff, enjoyed the opportunity to focus on the caring aspects of their role, and patients and family members seemed to appreciate the recognition of their needs. It was not clear, however, to what extent the appreciation of these aspects was due to the contrast with previous experiences or to their own inherent value.

The key aspects of palliative care—communication and open awareness and the concept of 'total pain'—as outlined in Chapter 2 are explored in the following chapters.

CHAPTER 5
Multi-dimensional care

Introduction

This chapter considers multi-dimensional care and how this is enacted through multi-disciplinary team working. Multi-disciplinary team working presents considerable challenges, both personal and professional. For some professionals, particularly nurses, these challenges may be part of the motivation for working in palliative care. Public perceptions of the roles of team members such as doctors, chaplains and social workers also present challenges to the working of the model of care. All professionals within the team work within the same philosophy of care, and for some there is considerable overlapping between professional roles. Others, such as doctors, perceive themselves to have a more defined clinical role. How the roles of core team members are defined and understood by the professionals and the public and the degree to which they overlap and share roles are explored in this chapter. Other staff in the organisation, for instance care assistants, administration and kitchen staff, work formally and informally to support the work of the core team, and their roles and their own perceptions of these roles are considered.

Communication is a core aspect of palliative care. Communication between team members is formally conducted through weekly meetings—multi-disciplinary meetings which review patients in the care of the service, and psychosocial meetings which focus on psychosocial problems in either a particular or general sense. In addition, communication between patients, family members and professional staff is also managed through family meetings held frequently at the hospice. These meetings and their outcomes are explored in this chapter.

Dealing with people

The two key aspects of palliative care—communication and 'total pain'—are perceived as separate but intrinsically interwoven. For professional staff, understanding and addressing the complex needs of patients and family members is facilitated through an emphasis and focus on the person rather than the illness.

> *'We treat people as a person whereas in other areas of medicine we treat them as the illness they have and not how that affects them as a person.'* (Margaret, doctor)

The focus on the person rather than the illness, highlighted in Margaret's remarks above, is at the core of palliative care. This focus is in contrast to other areas of health care and consequently entails a number of tasks that can often be avoided in other health care settings.

One of the central tasks of palliative care professionals, in their view, is to help people 'deal with the fact that they are dying', which often involves addressing uncomfortable and difficult issues about death and dying with patients and their family members.

> *'Part of what we do is helping people deal with the fact that they are dying. Not making them happy about it but helping people deal with the fact that they are dying. If you lose the fact that somebody needs to help people deal with the fact that they are dying, and hospices and palliative care are the people who do it now, if we don't do it, nobody else will do it. It is sad so it is easier to move off, it would be much easier for staff to say "We'll bring you in and sort out your bowels and you go home again", it would be much easier to go that road than the road of dealing with dying.'* (Sheila, doctor)

Karen, a nurse, felt that although communication and teamwork feature strongly in the 'language' of palliative care, these are, in practice, core aspects. Working with people at a deeper level than in other areas of health care also engaged practitioners at a deeper level, which could be personally demanding. Others, particularly nursing and chaplaincy staff, echoed this view.

> *'Communication skills and teamwork, ... it is so essential to palliative care and at a level that is much deeper than anywhere else because you are working very closely with people's deeper emotions and belief systems and that affects your own beliefs too.'* (Karen, nurse)

Multi-disciplinary team working

Within the multi-disciplinary team staff worked within a shared philosophy of care, and while each profession brought particular expertise to the team, the type of relationships that professionals had with the patient and family members was different.

Almost without exception, the professional staff in this study welcomed multi-disciplinary working. For some, particularly nurses, it was a welcome departure from previous experiences in other health care settings and was a compelling reason to continue working in palliative care. For the nursing staff, working within a multi-disciplinary team gave a broader perspective on the work they were doing and helped promote a sense of greater equality with other disciplines, in theory at least.

> *'It's brilliant, you know, they are always there... so there is a broader picture, because when you're a nurse you can sort of get focused in on symptoms... It's much different, it's just so much more on an equal level that, at least you know you can chat away and they'll listen to your opinions.'* (Lorraine, nurse)

Doctors, too, appreciated the input and expertise of some of the other professions, particularly the psychological viewpoint of social work.

> *'Working alongside people is a very useful learning tool. I would have no experience in working closely with, say, social workers or people coming from a more psychological viewpoint. You would have been aware of it but you didn't have the interactions on a day-to-day basis, which we now have, so I would think I would have learnt hugely from that and from that approach... as a team we have developed along the way.'* (Peter, doctor)

The multi-disciplinary team working, as part of this model of care, involves all team members working within a shared philosophy of care in response to the needs of patients and families. This approach requires, in theory, that team members engage with patients and families at the deep level that Karen talked about.

> *'The dogma of palliative care is that you try and be all things to all people and that you try and give some spiritual care, be you doctor, nurse or whatever. That you carry all these hats.'* (Peter, doctor)

Team working

Although the multi-disciplinary team approach is part of the model of palliative care, the way in which this aspect of the model worked in St Theresa's seemed to reflect a more traditional adherence to professional roles than may be the case in other cultures. Peter remarked that some of the staff who had worked in other countries found the Irish way of working difficult.

> *'The people who have found the Irish way difficult are people who have worked abroad for a while and come back.'* (Peter, doctor)

Staff who had worked within palliative care in other countries considered that, in spite of recent advancements, some aspects still lagged behind developments elsewhere, particularly the understanding of multi-disciplinary team working.

> *'I was surprised to find here on some levels there is a lot of advancements but on other levels we seem to be still back in the 1950s...in the layers of bureaucracy, I mean it takes forever to get anything done... and people are very conscious of their titles and their roles. You know, "That's my turf and you don't overstep". I think maybe there is a greater openness and maybe a teamwork approach [elsewhere]. When I say team, there is a recognition and acceptance that some roles overlap and that is okay.'* (Emer, nurse)

Emer felt that some of the practice issues, such as patient charts, really showed that a different view of team working prevailed in the hospice.

> *'There are different practice issues too. We only had one patient chart and everybody charted on it. The doctor, the nurse, the physiotherapist, the occupational therapist, whoever, everybody charted on it. Here I see separate charts and I wonder why. If there is one team, why is that? The view of teamwork seems to be quite different.'* (Emer, nurse)

Another example of professionals working within more traditional roles was an observation by Joan on the contribution of chaplains within the team. The role of the team members is more fully explored in the following chapter, but Joan felt that the chaplains retained something of the confessional aspects of the traditional role, were less inclined to share information about the details of the patient and seemed to keep the input into the multi-disciplinary meetings at a more abstract level.

> *'There is perhaps a little more privacy with the chaplains; they are much less inclined to tell you any of what they are talking about with people. The chaplain will say they are working with this person or seeing this person and they do have quite a few issues, spiritual issues, that are being resolved or they want to look at and that's going well or we are having a bit of trouble. But doesn't tell us the detail ... it's more abstract.'* (Joan, social worker)

Professional roles

Doctors, nurses, social workers and chaplains comprised the core team members at St Theresa's, although the composition of the core team may differ in other hospices and is dependent on available resources and organisational structures. Each professional discipline brought its own professional expertise to the team, so within this model the traditional roles of the team members were still the same: doctors and nursing staff looked after the control of physical symptoms, social workers were involved with the patient and the family, and chaplains concerned themselves with spiritual issues. Nevertheless, the team approach to care and the remit of multi-dimensional care led to overlaps between some of these roles, for instance social work and chaplaincy or chaplaincy and nursing. The team approach and the multi-dimensional focus provided considerable information about patients and family members, and the inclusion of the family within the remit of care also led to professional staff, particularly nursing staff and social workers, managing information and communication between patients and the family.

While the model offered the opportunity for professional staff to overlap and possibly extend their traditional roles, not all patients and family members accepted or welcomed this. The professional staff of the core team, with the exception of nursing, sometimes encountered preconceptions of their role that challenged the working of the model. In spite of these challenges, a team approach provided the opportunity to develop strategies for the delivery of care and evaluation of patient and family needs. The professional roles of the team members and the challenges to the roles are explored below.

Doctors

For the medical staff in the study, the focus on people rather than illness was a defining feature of palliative care and a major attraction. They felt that palliative care offered the opportunity to make a real difference to the quality of life of patients and their family members and this was a source of satisfaction.

> *'You diagnose an incurable cancer but there are a lot of problems and that was where I got an interest in what can you do with people that you can't cure but have a lot of problems.... And I would have always had an interest in people in a broad sense, an interest in people rather than an interest in diseases.'* (Sheila, doctor)

For Peter, the type of relationship that nurses often developed with patients was the attraction.

> *'I was drawn more and more towards it, towards talking to people. I had always done a lot of talking to people and always felt frustrated by my inability to do things for them. I always felt the nurses had a better time than we had.'* (Peter, doctor)

Preconceptions

The motivation for becoming involved in palliative care may reflect a desire for a more personal relationship with patients than was traditionally the case between doctors and patients; however, the perceptions of patients and family members seemed to remain within a more traditional form of this relationship model. This may have been due somewhat to the generally elderly profile of patients who, as Margaret remarked, have had a lifetime's experience of dealing with doctors and much of this experience has been negative.

> *'People have had fifty, sixty, eighty years' experience of doctors before and a recent example was a man, you know, we were talking away and he says "You know, well in the other hospital they would only stay five minutes", why are you still here nearly... They are not used, people sitting and having the time.'* (Margaret, doctor)

Patients sometimes interacted differently with doctors than with nursing staff.

> *'When the doctor is coming to see them, the patients gather up every ounce of strength that they have and they behave differently. "The doctor is coming". I have often had patients who maybe had a very restless night, had an awful lot of pain, talked to me a lot about their pain and the doctor would come and make rounds and I would say "She had a very bad night and she is having a lot of pain and I think we need to change the medication". Then he would go in and say "Hello, how are you today"? "Oh I'm fine thanks". "Did you sleep well"? "Not bad" .'* (Emer, nurse)

While the palliative care model provided a different approach, the stereotypical perceptions of doctors held by the patients and family members, for instance as belonging to particular social classes or the type of care that the doctors provided, were used on occasion by doctors and other professional staff to achieve particular objectives.

> *'I am a doctor and before anything is ever said that is putting me in people's minds somewhere, be it socially, be it level of care, the type of care, whatever. That puts me in a box... that may not be a bad thing, we use it sometimes.'* (Margaret, doctor)

Utilising these preconceptions also included using the authority traditionally vested in the medical profession.

> *'It's part of it, to the patients it's still a major one, a lot of them would listen to the doctor rather than the non-medical staff. You have to ask the doctor to say it because then they will say "The doctor said"... there is that group of people always, they don't feel that anyone else has the same authority.'* (Joan, social worker)

Social workers

With the inclusion of the family as part of the remit of care, the social aspects of care and family issues are the concerns of the social workers. At St Theresa's the relationship with the family continued after the death of the family member, and social workers were involved in the bereavement and after-care of the family.

The social work service at the hospice was a voluntary one, unlike other health care settings, such as hospitals, where discharge from the service may be dependent on a resolution of difficulties. Colm, one of the social workers at St Theresa's, told me that while the opportunity was offered to patients and families to address 'issues', this was always a choice. If they 'fail' to engage with this service, however, the patient may die without any of these issues being resolved.

> *'It's a voluntary role we have, we don't have any statutory rights, and we will offer families opportunities to address issues. However, families always have the choice whether to engage with any of what we offer and with the interdisciplinary nature of the work, a lot of psychosocial care is given to families and patients. But they exercise choice at every stage. In a hospital if there is a discharge date set, people have much less freedom to engage or disengage. Whereas here if they fail to engage, then the patient may die without any of that work being done but in reality they have a choice never to take up the service.'* (Colm, social worker)

While part of the work of social workers within this model involved addressing family issues, Kevin, another social worker at St Theresa's, saw the role as providing an outside view and a sounding board for patients and family members to 'rehearse' talking about death and dying without encountering the full emotional impact of family responses. Kevin saw this as enabling patients and family members to find solutions in ways that were appropriate for them.

> *'If they can be allowed to talk to someone outside the family about fears they may have because they may be unable to express it initially to other family members, they see how upset other family members are. If they can have, if you like a trial run nearly, with someone outside and then go back to the family or maybe work on strategies with the outsider about how to deal with it within the family, I think those are very important factors.'* (Kevin, social worker)

Problematic perceptions

Just as the doctors in the hospice found that patients and families often had past negative experiences of medical staff that shaped current perceptions, a similarly negative view of social workers was held by some families. Marie, one of the home care nurses, talked about a negative perception of the role of social workers: 'He is going to take your kids away, you have a problem immediately' (Marie, par. 66). Some families, according to Marie, had a view that once the social worker was involved, the family became a 'problem family.' This perception was problematic for the professional staff, and Marie talked about judging, in some cases, whether a chaplain who had a 'nice gentle way' and who could give Holy Communion was a better approach; this approach meant that problems or difficulties were not made explicit and sidestepped the difficulties about the involvement of the social worker.

> *'Sometimes if you are talking to somebody and you say a social worker they automatically think problems, "You think I have a problem", when sometimes if it is very gentle and they are not very definite about something, pastoral care can sometimes be a nicer way of broaching the subject with them. You know, a social worker is more definitely, counselling, definite problems where if it is someone that is just in a bit of distress and doesn't know what they are doing about it we have a chaplain who'll give you Holy Communion. It is a nice gentle way of dealing with it and it will just help them on their road without making such a definite statement of, you've got a problem, you need to deal with it.'* (Marie, nurse)

Marie also talked, in one instance, about working out an overall strategy which involved an initial visit from a chaplain with a further visit from a social worker when the patient had 'got used to talking'.

> *'In the conversation you get a feel, oh a social worker would be great here. But when you sit down and talk to them you think, well, hold on, you know, maybe we'll go gently and maybe if they go and see the chaplain they get used to talking but maybe then the social worker might come in later on and there might be a way of getting around that.'* (Marie, nurse)

Nurses

Nursing involves both clinical practice and a caring role, and within the palliative care model the caring aspect of nursing is more emphasised than in a curative model. For many of the nurses in the study, the motivation for becoming involved in palliative care was the opportunity and time to focus on caring for the patient. The caring role of nursing which the palliative care model supports also fits with the public perception of nursing and may be the reason why, of all the professions involved in the team, there seemed to be no negative preconceptions of the nursing staff by patients and family members.

> *'It's just because you've got so much time to deal with people and the whole atmosphere is different to general nursing. In general nursing if you were dealing with somebody you were constantly having to walk away from them and looking over your shoulder saying "I'll be back" and "I'm sorry, I'll come back to you in a few minutes"and knowing in your heart and soul most of the time you'd never get back to them. And knowing that people needed, they needed attention and you just didn't have the time to do it, once the physical stuff was done there was no time left. So I suppose the fact that you've got so much time here and everybody is open to you taking as much time as you want and the team is really flexible.'* (Fiona, nurse)

The emphasis on the caring aspects of nursing rather than on specifically caring for terminally ill people was the attraction for some of the nurses working in palliative care.

> *'I think a lot of people that are in palliative care have been through the hospital system, got fed up, and think there has to be another way of working. There's no mystery to palliative care, I think it's just the care that a lot of people would like to give universally to patients.'* (Catherine, nurse)

Although the remit of palliative care includes the family, nurses, in this study, saw their role as primarily caring and being an advocate for the patient.

> *'That is where we come in; we have to be an advocate for the patient.'* (Christine, nurse)

Managing potential conflicts

The issue of patient advocacy was a complex one, however. Although the priority for the nursing staff was the patient, in some cases it was difficult for nurses to manage the potential conflict between the patient's wishes and the wishes of family members; this in turn sometimes influenced the relationship between the nursing staff and the patients.

> *'There were issues a few weeks ago about a patient that didn't want to see a certain person and there was always talk of advocacy and stuff like that and on the one hand they were saying, you are advocate for the patient so I would say yes, the family are very important but your priority is to the patient. Your number one is the patient and you want to make them comfortable and keep them happy. On the other hand, legally, we actually can't stop somebody coming in, we could advise them not to come in but we actually couldn't physically stop somebody coming in. So it's all sorts of issues like that, that if somebody says to you I don't want to see so-and-so and then you say back to them, well I can't actually physically stop them coming in, and there are ideas of trust and other issues flying around the place.'* (Catherine, nurse).

The nursing role seemed to involve a considerable amount of managing, in particular of family members in relation to the patient but also managing the family in the physical space of the hospice. These aspects of the nursing role are considered in more detail in the following chapter under 'Managing space and social ties'.

Chaplains

Traditionally the role of chaplaincy within health care settings has been a sacramental role. This role, within palliative care in particular, has now evolved into one of accompaniment in addition to some sacramental duties. As the role has changed there are now overlaps between some health care professionals, such as nursing and social work.

Chaplains in Ireland complete CPE training to qualify as a chaplain. With the introduction of this training, nuns and lay people are now eligible for chaplaincy posts that in the past were the domain of ordained ministers. Nevertheless, chaplains are trained by religious foundations and within particular religious traditions. Non-ordained ministers may not administer sacraments such as confession or anointing with oils (the Sacrament of the Sick), and therefore for some chaplains it falls short of a full sacramental role.

The chaplaincy team at St Theresa's consisted of two religious sisters, Pauline and Bernadette, and Father Michael. Church of Ireland (Anglican Church) patients were cared for by Reverend David, the local Church of Ireland minister. Patients from other faiths, such as one patient who belonged to the Russian Orthodox Church, were cared for by ministers from their own church.

Father Michael conducted Mass every day in the hospice and also visited patients with Holy Communion every day. Pauline and Bernadette were less involved in a sacramental role, although they did administer Holy Communion, but they felt that their role was more one of accompaniment, with the patient in particular. This role placed them in a very close and personal relationship with some patients, which they felt was very demanding and had a different starting position from the sacramental role of chaplaincy.

> *'The old idea was to come and give the sacraments and get people to pray and all that. I think you don't begin with religion, you begin with the spiritual, it's beginning where the person is.'* (Pauline, chaplain)

Chaplaincy also involved a religious perspective; however, Bernadette felt that this new starting place allowed for the exploration of the nature of the religious perspective and practice of the patient.

> *'Going initially with a patient, you don't really know what the religious practice of this patient may have been. Even though they may be the same religion as ourselves, they may have practised their religion in a very different way.'* (Bernadette, chaplain)

While chaplains saw their role as accompaniment without preconceptions and judgement, in many instances patients and family members did have preconceptions and negative past experiences of the Church and representatives of the Church that hampered interaction.

> *'Father Michael would go around and just generally say hello to people and just suss them out and see where they are coming from. And this man, when he saw him, said "I want nothing to do with that man" and you know he didn't want anything to do with the chaplains for his whole duration of his time in here. Again, he put it down to, he had had bad experiences along the way and he was going to die his own way, he wasn't going to have anything from the Church.'* (Bernadette, chaplain)

An accompanying role

Pauline and Bernadette, because they were not ordained ministers and therefore had a limited sacramental role, talked a lot about their role as being one of 'accompaniment'; they saw a number of aspects to this, such as listening to concerns and resolving difficulties—both temporal and spiritual—that the patient may have.

> *'Maybe in listening then it allows them to look at issues and maybe come up with some steps of what to do or decisions, to what area to go.'* (Bernadette, chaplain).

The act of listening and being present with patients rather than focusing on tasks and 'doing' was, of itself, a spiritual experience.

> *'Because in doing things, maybe you can avoid what the real thing can be and it's trying to help the person uncover or find what it is that they are so upset or worried about or it may be something from their past that they are finding difficult, it is enabling the person to express that without judgement,*

> *with compassion. I think that is what as a chaplain I would be trying to do but I have no right to judge anybody about anything. I treat that person with compassion. I suppose if I can do that and give this person time, to be present to them, in the best way that I can, for whatever the issue is; it may not be a spiritual issue at all. But in the telling of it and being able to be there with that person that is a spiritual experience.'* (Pauline, chaplain)

Both the chaplains felt that working with patients and family members in this way was personally very demanding and required a high level of reflection.

> *'You know where you are yourself, in your spirituality, in your reflections, in a way, reflecting on what you are doing and not all the time rushing and flying and hyped up. But you have to find some kind of a stillness in yourself, in your own spiritual journey before you can be with someone in a spiritual dimension.'* (Pauline, chaplain)

This reflection involved a constant questioning of what the patient actually wanted and needed.

> *'When I go in to a person I would never offer to pray with them. I don't go in to, you know, pour prayers down, I go in to be with the person. I try to ascertain how that person wants me to be with him or her, which can be difficult at times and there can be an awful lot of questioning in me. Am I forcing myself or does this person really need or want me to be here?'* (Bernadette, chaplain)

Pauline spoke to me about often feeling very vulnerable in these relationships and especially when going into a room to see a patient, as, unlike the nursing staff, she had nothing to 'do' and could only bring herself.

> *'I go in to somebody and I can't bring anything. I can only bring myself. The nurse can bring in the tablets.'* (Pauline, chaplain)

Although the chaplaincy role can be a solitary one, chaplaincy staff felt supported by colleagues and felt a shared sense of responsibility for the spiritual welfare of patients and family members.

> *'I found since I came here that I am not alone ... I always feel supported by the nurses especially and the doctors and I feel the spirituality of the people does not depend totally on me.'* (Bernadette, chaplain)

There was also a support provided by handing the work over to a higher power and a sense of being a mediator rather than the person who is doing the work.

> *'I go into the oratory in the morning and I don't stay long now, this is when I come into work and I just put the whole day in the hands of the Lord and I ask him to guide me just to be the way that people need me to be. I think that carries me because okay I have to put my best into it but there is somebody else with me, you know it is not just me.'* (Bernadette, chaplain)

Overlapping roles

The chaplains did not consider the role of accompanying patients as being exclusive to chaplaincy and encouraged staff to also engage with this role.

> *'I would be up there saying to all the staff. It is not just for me. I might have more expertise in the whole thing, you know to go in and talk to people about their spiritual lives and the prayer and the pastoral thing. But that whole thing of presence and being with people, I think all of the staff here are very tuned into that.'* (Pauline, chaplain)

Nurses often developed a level of intimacy and trust with patients that touched on aspects of the chaplaincy role of accompaniment. Some of the nurses, however, especially those who associated spiritual care closely with religious care, were uncomfortable with this perceived overlap and felt out of their depth when patient concerns became matters of existential concerns or difficulties with religious belief and practice.

> *'This one particular lady, I felt at such a loss because really I didn't know where to go. I felt that she needed much more than I could give, like she*

> *was talking about the afterlife and things like that and as much as I would consider myself quite spiritual it is very difficult if you are talking to a patient. You are very conscious of putting your views on someone else and in the end... I just waited and I said that I really think you need to talk to someone... and I don't think that I am the right one. So I did refer her back to the chaplains.'* (Geraldine, nurse)

In contrast, Catherine, who had previously worked in a nurse-led service without the services of a chaplain, was quite comfortable talking about spiritual issues with patients.

> *'Just because there is a spiritual issue you don't automatically have to get the chaplain, you can talk about it.'* (Catherine, nurse)

Patients, however, also chose whom they spoke to about their concerns. Although the philosophy of care suggests that all members of staff can talk with patients about all aspects of concern, Margaret felt that patients put professionals into boxes.

> *'They are not going to talk to me about spiritual issues, and ... whether we like it or not some of us would be labelled and while we try and put across the idea that any one of us would talk to them about any issue as best we can, people put you in boxes.'* (Margaret, doctor)

Margaret also felt that the way in which she or her fellow medical colleagues spoke about spiritual concerns probably revealed a lack of expertise and therefore patients would not always be comfortable in talking about spiritual concerns with medical staff.

> *'When I ask somebody if religion or spirituality is important, even the way I ask the questions shows that I wouldn't be great at opening this area up.'* (Margaret, doctor)

There were also overlaps between the roles of chaplains and social workers, as indicated earlier. In the in-patient unit, with a chaplain and social worker present every day, the interaction between the professional staff was more fluid, whereas in home care the intervention of one or other of the professionals needed to be made more explicit as the visits were pre-arranged.

The decision concerning which professional to send depended on individual need and appropriateness, and this was assessed by either the home care doctor or nurse. Peter outlined how this decision might be reached; for instance, when there were issues of deep loss or tragedy it was felt that the chaplain might provide comfort or consolation, and sometimes a male or female presence was also a consideration.

> *'Sometimes it's totally clear issues, a person might want somebody to come and pray with them, that's clear, like the sacraments brought to them, that's clear, are angry with God and they can't pray, that's very clear-cut. When it becomes issues of loss and past life tragedies that seem to be invading the spirit of somebody, I have a difficulty in knowing which to call sometimes. And sometimes, being honest, on our own team we have male and female in the roles and sometimes I think this is more for a man, more for a woman, you know. Because I would see an overlap in some aspects of the roles but obviously the pastoral person would bring a dimension of religion.'* (Peter, doctor)

Supporting roles

The professional roles of doctors, nurses, social workers and chaplains formed a core multi-disciplinary team working in the hospice. Care assistants, administration and kitchen staff worked to support the professional staff in their care of patients and their families. These roles were often blurred; some, such as kitchen staff and administration staff, had no apparent direct role in relation to patients and family members, although in practice this did occur informally. Care assistants, a relatively new post within the health care structure in Ireland, had a direct role with patients and families.

Care assistants

The role of the care assistant was, according to the professional nurses, to look after the feeding, toileting, mobility and general hygiene aspects of care. Care assistants were assigned a mentor from among the nursing staff and had the opportunity to raise difficulties or questions with this person. The care assistants seemed to occupy a peripheral role in relation to the team. In some instances care assistants attended a multi-disciplinary meeting, but this seemed to be only when they had a direct relationship with a patient and could provide information for the team; more frequently they attended a psychosocial meeting, as these meetings were often presented as case-studies and were seen as an educational opportunity for staff.

Care assistants, in looking after the physical tasks of caring for patients, were generally in close and intimate proximity to patients. This position offered the opportunity to observe patients, although this may not be explicitly understood by patients.

> *'We give them their breakfast and we might have to feed somebody, depends if they can't feed themselves ... Or else you might just sit and you are letting on that you are just sitting there and you are there watching them.'* (Isobel, care assistant)

Although the position of care assistants in health care in Ireland was relatively new, some of the nursing staff appreciated their input and skill. Noirin, one of the nurses in the in-patient unit, felt that this contribution was often overlooked.

> *'A couple of the care assistants are fantastic with the patients and why that isn't utilised I'll never know, one girl in particular is excellent with the patients, I enjoy working with her, she is brilliant with the patients. I don't think they are always remembered, you know if somebody dies, the care assistants work with you as well, they might be sitting with the patient and that's not always remembered.'* (Noirin, nurse)

Other nurses, however, were concerned about the lack of training and queried the degree to which care assistants could manage some of the professional aspects of care, such as dealing with family dynamics in the in-patient unit, the type of information to give to family members and the importance of confidentiality.

'It worries me a little bit, the level of training, not the personalities. People working in a supermarket one week and then at a psychosocial meeting the next week.... I see a lot of conversations going on with care assistants and relatives and care assistants and patients and I just wonder to myself sometimes what the level of professionalism in that conversation is because the patients and the relatives are talking and perceive this person as a professional a lot of the time, in a uniform.' (Laura, nurse)

Administration and kitchen staff

Administration staff and kitchen staff were included in this study; these workers provided formal and informal support for the core team. Almost without exception, the staff felt that by working in this setting they contributed to the care of patients and their families.

'For me it's not the wage package that I am going to get at the end of the week, it's actually being in here, you are working for the patient, you feel you are helping the patients.' (Monica, administration)

For some of the staff, for instance Elizabeth, who worked at reception and came into contact with families, there were opportunities to make a direct contribution to the welfare and care of people.

'She was standing there just in reception and ... she had one child in her arms and the other pulling at her and she was just distraught and ... we were actually trying to amuse the children.' (Elizabeth, administration)

Although these members of staff were not the professional carers, they did manage aspects of care. Helen related a time when, on answering a phone call, she encountered a very distressed person who on hearing the holding music on the telephone had been reminded of phone calls made to the hospice when her husband was alive. Helen stayed on the phone to this lady and talked with her about her distress.

'I just happened to take this call, the phone was ringing and I just picked it

> *up. And the woman was crying... before I said anything, she had been put on hold and it was the music. She recalled that she would ring her husband daily and ... the music would come on. She almost anticipated that she was going to hear his voice on the other end and instead it was mine.'* (Helen, administration)

Carmel, who worked in the canteen, expressed concern and empathy for family members whom she encountered; she told me about wanting to do something to make things better for them but sometimes felt frustrated that she could only make them a sandwich, although she put a lot of care into doing this and felt that this was her contribution to their care.

> *'You see family members coming down to the restaurant and you see tears and you see pain in their eyes and there is nothing you can do bar make them a sandwich. That sometimes gets to me... It's the only way I can help them and if that's all I can do, do it right is my attitude.'* (Carmel, kitchen staff)

The kitchen staff provided a level of informal support for nursing staff that encompassed a degree of sensitivity to and awareness of their needs that may not have been immediately apparent. Carmel told me about always making sure that there was enough variety in the menu in the restaurant.

> *'I always think that if the nurses are looking at the same food that the patients are having, there is an association there. Whereas it is their break time and there should be no associations, they are on their free time, time to cut off, for half an hour or an hour when they do not have to think of the patient.'* (Carmel, kitchen staff)

A sense of uncertainty

Although working in the service gave the staff a sense of contributing to patient care, many of the administration staff felt very much on the periphery and uncertain about the appropriate level of contact with patients and their family members. Jean had dealings with some families prior to admission and she talked about the uncertainty of how to deal with family members once they came into the hospice.

> *'I would deal with people who come in and want to get their family member into the hospice, I would maybe organise nursing staff to show them around. A person will phone me every day and will say "Have you got a bed for my Dad, my husband or whatever?" And you are talking to them so you get to know them for maybe a few weeks and then they come in and you see them on the corridor and I would say "Hello, how are you?" But I'm not sure whether I should be going over to them and saying how are you? And that role is not clear.'* (Jean, administration)

Jean talked specifically about a case where she did have contact with the son of a patient and was uncertain how to behave towards the person when she met him in the hospice. Her uncertainty about the appropriateness of contact with family members once they have come into the hospice seemed to stem from not being the 'professional' carers of patients and family members.

> *'I had had a particular case where I had dealt with this guy a lot about his Dad, he was a really lovely man and when his Dad came in, I would just say "Hi, how are you?" in the corridor and he must have thought it strange that I am not saying how are things? But I didn't feel that was my job to do that, or that wasn't defined so subsequently his Dad died and the following week he rang and he said "Look, there is just a message on Mum's answering machine and she's confused, she doesn't know whether it came in just before my Dad died or is it a new message". So I said that's fine, I'll check that out, but the interesting thing was that he came back to me, I was the contact. So that is a bit fuzzy, we are the poor relations, we are not the "'professionals".'* (Jean, administration)

Many of the administration staff talked about a 'line you can't cross', although they were not quite sure what this line was and where it was situated. Susan felt uncomfortable when a patient came directly to her to talk about something that concerned him, because she felt that this was not her role and that the patient should have been talking to a professional counsellor.

> *'I have to be careful what I say to people, I mean there are nurses, there*

> *are counsellors, I am just in administration, there is a line and there are certain things you can't say, you have to be very careful. I can be comforting to people to a degree and they often come to me and say, especially if I know them from outside, "Nice to see a familiar face" and that's fine. But there is a certain line you can't cross, I had one instance of a man and he had a problem and I don't know why but he zoned in on me. He came one day and he was very upset and he started to tell me something and I said "There are counsellors if you would like", "No, no", he said, "I don't want to talk to them, I need to tell you".'* (Susan, administration)

Although the staff did not see themselves as professional carers, they were aware of and did manage aspects of the professional role such as confidentiality.

> *'Confidentiality is a huge thing here because there is still a kind of stigma about being here and dying and that people mightn't even want neighbours to know where they are. And people can be just private and not want, even people phoning, you have to be very careful. Someone might ring and say "A neighbour of mine, I don't see her around but I believe she is very bad and she is in there" and I just say "Gosh, I'll just put you through to the nurses, they will know the patients". Put her through and let the nurses deal with it, you know that particular patient didn't want any of her neighbours to know where she was or to be coming visiting.'* (Elizabeth, administration)

Many of the administration staff talked to me about how working in the hospice, no matter how remote the contact with patients and their families was, affected them.

> *'You are still working in that environment, you know, and more often I think there can be a sense around the place that something is going on...you would get a feeling or vibe that there was a large family or if there was a young person on the ward, or a young family with children. And you are very aware, you are working away but you are listening into, you are nearly tuning in and can nearly hear things. Children's voices or children crying. You are doing your work but it does impact on you, it does impact on you.'* (Helen, administration)

Staff also felt guarded about saying where they worked because working in the hospice had increased their own awareness of the impact of death and bereavement on people, and this made them cautious in their conversations with people outside of the hospice. Jean told me about casual conversations with other people and how careful she felt she had to be.

> *'If I say where I work people ask me am I affected by being here. Because you know everybody knows somebody who's been here. One woman talked in particular about home care and how great it was but I am always conscious about what I say. I don't know what these people have been through. I don't know if they are going to be in. If they have had bereavement, you have to be so careful about how you talk about death and where you work with people because it has such an impact on people or it touches something within them.'* (Jean, administration)

Modes of interaction

Core team members attended the multi-disciplinary and psychosocial meetings. The multi-disciplinary meetings evolved from staff update meetings, which are the norm in health care settings, in which the information about each patient and family was reviewed. Psychosocial meetings specifically looked at psychosocial and spiritual issues, which seemed to be the non-medical issues. At some meetings the focus was on problems with specific patients and families; at other times the focus was more abstract and prompted by issues such as family violence or difficult family dynamics that were impacting on the care of a patient.

Multi-disciplinary meetings

During multi-disciplinary meetings medical updates were established first; information was also provided by nurses, social workers and chaplains in turn, although not necessarily in this order. Staff liked the multi-disciplinary approach as it allowed a fuller and more comprehensive picture to be drawn of the patient and the family. In some instances a social worker or chaplain had a close relationship with a patient and their insight was considered very useful.

> *'Things might be brought up because they are considered relevant, especially if the person seems unhappy. Then the input would be from who*

> *has got to know the person well, who's looped in, who's relating, it could be the chaplain, it was in one particular case. The chaplain did it all, had the trust of that patient through a spiritual perspective. They prayed together and somehow the chaplain was able to make an opening and the patient was able to respond to something that happened to her when she was younger, something to do with conscience. Being free of a secret and then was offered the opportunity of being able to resolve that in real ways, not just pray but in real ways. Now at first, she did not want to stir that up, "No I don't want to think about it" and then saying "No I won't speak to him" and after a few weeks it was "I want to". The chaplain facilitated all that, it could be one of the doctors, really teamwork. It's definitely not handed to someone who doesn't know the person.'* (Joan, social worker)

Occasionally the picture was more fragmented, and small pieces of information from different perspectives were drawn together to present a more coherent picture.

> *'Sometimes I would arrive at a meeting with a sense that we know very little about what is going on for this patient and a lot of other people arriving individually at the meeting feeling exactly the same, their interactions have been limited or there has been a breakdown in communication. When you sit down together you often find that putting the pieces together you have a much clearer sense of... a much bigger picture and you know it kind of assimilates all the aspects of patient care, physical concerns, emotional concerns, family concerns, spiritual concerns and it helps usually in generating ideas about how best to care for somebody.'* (Carol, doctor)

While these meetings may provide information for a larger, clearer picture of the patient and family, one of the nursing staff expressed concerns to me about the amount of information regarding patients and families that was discussed at these meetings.

> *'Sometimes I say to myself if this was me and my family, how would I feel? I know we work as a team but there are so many details of somebody's life and there are so many people there, I would worry about it a little bit.'* (Laura, nurse)

While the team approach suggests that each professional on the team has an equal contribution, at the time I conducted the research the medical information concerning the patient was always the first input of the meeting. When I spoke to Joan, the social worker, about how the meetings were organised, she assured me that while this information was addressed first because the doctors could read the symptoms and keep the patient pain-free, this did not mean that it was privileged, as within palliative care doctors acknowledge that a lot of pain is caused by emotional or spiritual problems.

> *'Medical is not supposed to be on top, yes, medical information, medical knowledge is not privileged but it has to be because they read the symptoms and keep people pain-free. But that's a simplistic thing because the doctors here constantly acknowledge that a lot of the pain is from emotional and spiritual problems and that is why we don't privilege the administering of drugs as much as normal hospitals.'* (Joan, social worker)

Nevertheless, the priority given to the medical perspective may more accurately reflect the traditional authority of this profession. A different view of the meeting was expressed by some of the nursing staff, who considered that, in spite of the team approach, the decisions were always made by the doctor who is present at the meeting.

> *'A group of disciplines sitting down but still the decision-maker is the doctor and the decision, that decision that is made is rarely influenced by what other people say.'* (Emer, nurse)

Family meetings

Communication with the patient and the family was also facilitated by the family meetings, which were generally held two or three times a week. The primary purpose of these meetings was seen as an exchange of information between the professional staff, the patient and the family members. These meetings were arranged as the need arose, needs being identified by the professional staff. Patients were included in the meeting, when they were well enough to attend, and the patient's permission for a meeting was required. When patients were too unwell to communicate their wishes about this, permission for the meeting was sought from the next of kin.

Ostensibly, the family meeting was a mechanism for keeping the family updated with the medical information and prognosis; however, the impetus for a family meeting seemed to arise when there were large numbers of family members or when there were family tensions present. A meeting was called in order to ensure that the family members were given the same information. A further need identified by staff was when there seemed to be unresolved issues present which were affecting the patient.

> *'The policy is that it has to enhance the patients' well-being or care or the families' well-being which is part of our care, in other words it's not just gossip. So it has to be something that maybe potentially will make a difference to the person being free of pain, physical discomfort, torment, emotional distress, being able to die well. And I have seen people unable to die, hang on till something resolves.'* (Joan, social worker)

Family meetings were seen as an important vehicle for the exchange of information between the family and the professional staff, which sometimes had a profound effect on the patient.

> *'It's an exchange of information. We have had dramatic revelations from families that have transformed that person's care so there is always that. Like we didn't know that, one woman had had a teenage pregnancy forty years before and the child had been adopted out in another country and this was what was tormenting her and nothing could seem to relieve her stress. One of the staff members knew somebody who did tracing in that country; by the time she died, she had not met the man, the person, but had spoken several times to him on the phone. Knew how he had been about his life and how he was and knew he didn't resent what she done and he was enormously pleased to have had the chance to find out why it had happened. She was a good woman and had had a good life, she learnt that he had had a good life and that information came from someone in the family, I don't suppose she would ever have told us.'* (Joan, social worker)

While the focus of the meetings was the exchange of information with a view to improving or enhancing care, Bernadette, one of the chaplains, felt that this way of trying to resolve problems was not always appropriate for the patient.

> *'We find sometimes at our meetings that you are saying there is something going on with that person, why won't she or he talk about it, and yet we have to say, well, how did he or she deal with it in the past. And often times, they didn't deal with it by talking about it, they solved it in their own way and it's trying to respect that. I think we have to be careful. ... We need to be critical about the way we deal with people so that we may hopefully meet them where they need to be met.'* (Bernadette, chaplain)

Summary

This chapter has considered the professional roles of the members of the core multi-disciplinary team in the care of patients and families. For the professional staff, this form of health care model—the focus on people rather than illness and the team working aspects—provided the opportunity to expand their traditional professional roles and to establish relationships with patients and family members, although resistance to this was sometimes encountered in the response of patients and families to professionals, particularly doctors and social workers.

The aim of providing holistic care for patients and family members was facilitated by multi-disciplinary and psychosocial meetings, which provided the opportunity for sharing and thus expanding the available information about patients and families in order to enhance care. Professional staff who had made a connection or established a relationship with patients and families often provided key information. Patients, however, chose whom they would talk to and rarely spoke with doctors concerning spiritual and other personal concerns.

Staff who worked in other areas of the hospice, such as administration and the kitchen, valued the opportunity to contribute to patient and staff care and provided informal support within the organisation. Although palliative care is focused on the person rather than illness, some of the staff felt uncertain about the appropriate level of contact with patients and family members as they were not the professional carers.

It would appear that in order to achieve the aims of the model of palliative care, i.e. the holistic care of patients and families, a relationship of some kind needs to be established in order for intimate and sensitive issues to be understood and addressed. Patients, however, chose with whom they had this relationship and it was not always with professional staff. The nature of these relationships and how they are shaped and influenced by the physical location of care is explored in the following chapter.

CHAPTER 6
Relationship and place

Introduction

Within palliative care the primary care relationship is that between the patient and palliative care professionals. There are, however, relationships between the palliative care professionals and the family and between the family members and the patients.

The level and form of communication are directly influenced by cultural norms of communication and family cultures. The family culture may fit easily with the culture and aims of palliative care and the values of the organisation, but this is not always the case. The management of these issues is dependent upon and influenced by the relationship between the patient, the family and the palliative care professionals, and this is explored in this chapter.

The relationships between palliative care professionals and patients and family members occur in different places: in the family home and in the hospice day care service and the in-patient unit. This chapter examines how place shapes the nature and management of these relationships.

The nature of the relationship

The primary focus of attention within palliative care is the patient and the patient's needs. Separating the patient from the family and the patient's needs from the needs of the family can be difficult, however, particularly in Irish culture, where these relationships are very much interwoven.

> *'The patient is the primary person that we are looking after and a great sensitivity [is needed] in respecting a patient's autonomy and asking patients' permission about who they share their information with. Who of the family that we speak to, particularly in Irish culture the patient would particularly want for you to talk to all their family and involve all their family.'* (Carol, doctor, par. 64)

Communication

A central feature of palliative care is an open awareness of death and dying and communication between the patient, the family and palliative care professionals. The degree to which there can be open awareness and communication is dependent to some extent on the existing culture of the family. A close match between the culture of the family and the culture of palliative care facilitated the implementation of palliative care in a manner that fitted well with its overall philosophy.

> '*Clearly for us from the point of view of looking after somebody and probably for the well-being of the patient and the family, the family that can talk about things openly and where things are open and above board would seem to us to be better.*' (Peter, doctor, par. 27)

The aims of palliative care, particularly, that of facilitating a 'good death' through open awareness and communication, are idealistic, and while this was understood by palliative care professionals as such, meeting situations within families that impeded the implementation of these aims created difficulties. For some palliative care professionals in this study, a less-than-open approach was problematic as it created a tension between the aims of the model, the underlying philosophy and the way in which these could be met.

> '*We have all different ethical stances, I mean we all want the good of people, but we want it differently too. I suppose we are as different as the patients we meet in many ways are... some people would find a situation where total honesty is somewhat compromised makes them feel that they are not able to carry out their job properly.*' (Peter, doctor, par. 38)

The point of balance

There are subtle differences between providing patient-focused care from the vantage point of the patient and the family on the one hand and providing patient-focused care from the vantage point of palliative care professionals on the other.

When the family culture of communication is at odds with the aims of palliative care, compromising the ideals of the palliative care model can make professionals uncomfortable. On the other hand, caring for the patient and the family from the perspective of palliative care—that is, pursuing open awareness—may hurt and distress some families, who may be uncomfortable with the ideas of open awareness and communication.

> '*The mother was the one initially that had tried to defend her husband from any bad news and the family saw that she was vindicated, that he had a "good death" without our information ... We have to take cognisance of that. I think that maybe they are right and we try to balance ourselves with that, but maybe sometimes they are right and maybe that is good for the person, I mean it's hard to imagine but maybe, maybe that is the right way for them ... I have met people afterwards who have said that they were very happy that they had done it that way; that they had saved their loved one suffering, mental suffering in some way. Now our argument was that they had shut the person off from talking about it, or the opportunity and that would be where we come from.*' (Peter, doctor, par. 29–36)

Getting this balance wrong resulted in increasing rather than decreasing family tensions and created distress for the family and difficulties for palliative care professionals.

> '*We talk about addressing people holistically and about being there for their family as well. If there are frightened families and frightened patients then part of our remit is to bring them together and facilitate that. It is a lot of work and people can get very hurt in it, they can get criticised, they can get phone calls back to work. There are risks in it and you know risks of being told you are wrong, risks of being told you have hurt somebody. You can make people very unhappy and you try your best not to.*' (Peter, doctor, par. 61)

Some of the social workers that I spoke to looked at the situation from the perspective of the family and seemed to adopt a flexible rather than a prescriptive approach. This helped to reconcile two potentially different perspectives and involved viewing the situation and seeing the difficulties from the perspective of the family while at the same time continuing to offer the facilities of the palliative care service.

> *'It's all very well to say "Oh this is how you should do it, this is the 'good death plan', a, b, c, d, you'll be fine". But in any stressful situation do I react in the most logical fashion or appropriate way? No, absolutely not. When I look at any family, or get to know any family, you get to see the other difficulties there, the other factors that you have to take into account. The other points that you have to consider when you are saying "Well, can we create a better situation here" is that no family wants to get it wrong, if there is a right and wrong, no family wants to do that. They all want to do what is best and they all strive to do that. Sometimes they are able to hear what we have to say and sometimes they are not, because of their own situation. I think all we can do as professionals is try and support them in their decisions, offer advice if they are seeking it but at the end of the day, we are offering it. If they choose not to take it or not able to take it for their own personal reasons because of their own circumstances, well I think we have to respect that and still continue to work with them.'* (Kevin, social worker, par. 56)

Locations of care

The palliative care services at St Theresa's included day care, home care and an in-patient unit. These settings shaped the relationships between the palliative care professionals and patients and family members and provided a variety of vantage points, and consequently different points of balance were required. The balance between the patient and family perspective and that of the professionals altered according to the location. Palliative care professionals were visitors when the patient was at home, and patients were visitors in the in-patient services.

Home care

In this setting, the position of palliative care professionals as visitors seemed clear, and those I spoke to were aware that their relationship with a patient and a family was one of visitor, and sometimes a very temporary visitor. As such the professional staff needed to fit in with the family and the patient, and as a result seemed to have less control over aspects such as open awareness and communication. The home care service engaged with the patient and the family at a level of need and involvement defined by the patient and the family.

> '*In the home you are on other people's, it's their home, it's not yours, so you go in as a professional to offer services but you have to be respectful of people's views and wishes and you have go around things gently.*' (Peter, doctor, par. 61)

Introducing the services of the hospice in the home was sometimes difficult; some families resisted palliative care as it meant there was no longer any cure, and there was a sense that allowing the palliative care professionals in the door allowed death in the door.

> '*There are a number of people who see that admitting us through the door is the admission that we are needed and the admission that death is coming and to some extent you are almost blamed for it, it's a kind of an entangled web.*' (Peter, doctor, par. 67)

The doctors in the home care service at St Theresa's were the first to visit the patient and the family at home. There was a degree of uncertainty about what kind of reception they would receive; in some cases this was open and straightforward, in others there was a sense of inching forward and trying to find out, tentatively, how much the family knew about the illness and the prognosis and what was the family's understanding about the palliative care services.

> '*There is of course the folklore that hospice means dying, and you edge your way into people's houses. Within our team, you see, we*

> *have these big discussions and a number of people feel that you should walk through the door and say "Hello, I am the doctor from St Theresa's, how are you, Mrs Jones." I don't go that way about things. I usually work my way in and by the time I am finishing I try and break where I come from. There are some situations where I walk straight in and say who I am and it's all open and that's fine. Where I am not sure I would edge my way in and sometimes you are on a winner, the family are all edgy, they want you to tell them but they don't know how it is going to go so you have got "Where are you from?". "We work in the community and we give palliative care, that is the control of symptoms, that's associated with your disease" and you go gingerly, you know it's all feel, feel. "And there is a team of workers, they are called the home care team, never heard of it? From ...", now that is enough a lot of the time not to go any further. So the nurses and a team itself from .... can be enough, for others it can mean not a thing. But for quite a lot they go "Ah" when you say the place.*' (Peter, doctor, par. 225)

Although the home care team members in this study suggested that some professionals felt that there should be complete openness about where they are from and what the service is about, nobody I spoke to actually expressed that view. Those I spoke with who worked in home care—nurses, doctors and social workers—felt that the position of professionals was one of visitors who had a responsibility to work within the existing family pattern, and to leave it intact for family members after the death.

> '*Let's say there has been an existing relationship for sixty years and they have this established pattern of communication within a family. What we are trying to do is help them within that existing pattern for the short time that we are involved without causing disruption and mayhem to that pattern, hopefully help them to adjust it a little so that they can deal more fully with their situation. But at the end of the day leave them intact because they have had this pattern for so long, after we are gone, they will still be there... the remaining members of the family still have to relate.*' (Kevin, social worker, par. 82)

Managing respect and autonomy

Underlying patient-focused care is the issue of respecting patient and family autonomy and supporting the family in the care of the dying person. These aspects can conflict with the palliative care way of 'doing things', and the right balance was hard to achieve as this was different in every situation and could also change over the period of time that the relationship between family and palliative care services existed. Peter talked about some families and patients who did not fit into an 'idealised model', and by implication it would appear that families and patients who engaged with the service at the final stages did not fit into this idealised model.

> '*Sometimes you go out kind of "fire brigading" at the end which is not ideal for us but then sometimes they can be amazingly grateful and you think that you had been there for six months, that's all they wanted, you know. They wanted you in for the last few days, the last, and they have managed the other bit in their own way and that's about empowering people as well. We would have this idealised model but people don't always fit into our way of doing things*.' (Peter, doctor, par. 73–5)

Part of this model is providing support at all levels, physical, emotional, social and spiritual, but not all families wanted or required this type of involvement. Sometimes a minimal involvement was due to the rapid progress of the terminal illness and a late referral to the service, but other families needed only a minimal level of clinical support and symptom management as they provided social and emotional support for the patient and family members themselves.

> '*It depends, you could see somebody last week and they could die very peacefully and have a very nice death and the family are fine, they are very thankful, and you might only see them once or twice. Last week I saw a patient on Friday, twice on Saturday, twice on Sunday and he died very early Monday morning and the family were very happy. He wanted to die at home and he died at home. You know, it is a lot to do with the support that he got so there is no set regime, and it is just being there for them when they want you.*' (Marie, nurse, par. 34)

Family, friends and the community in which patients lived sometimes provided the kind of support that is part of the palliative care model.

> '*I can see enormous strength from community. I had the experience of going into a block of flats where there was a young woman dying. ... It was in the morning time and there was somebody scrubbing the steps, her sister, she scrubbed the steps because I had come to see the patient. You could feel the sense in it that they were watching and waiting with this young woman who had lived there nearly all her life, that huge sense of the entire community almost like a village.*' (Peter, doctor, par. 19)

One of the home care nurses, Karen, talked about feeling very much a stranger when she arrived at a house to look after a patient with whom there had been no pre-existing relationship. This was an intimate family time, with family and friends present, and she felt uncomfortable; she spoke about spending the afternoon going in and out to the car, so that she could leave the family to look after their mother while at the same time being on hand in case they needed her.

> '*I felt very much a stranger. This is a very intimate family time ... I never met the patient although I was with her in her last few hours ... so most of my time was taken up with trips to and from the house to the car ... There were photographs of her in the house. They were around the room and people said things about her. I think the thing about somebody being at home is that you can get a group of people that know a person very well, they will sit around and recall stories. There was something very supportive for them all to be able to share those memories and there is a support in it almost like a wake situation.*' (Karen, nurse, par. 28–30)

Caring for the dying person at home provided an opportunity to sustain or develop an intimacy between the dying person and family carers, a level of intimacy that may not be possible for family carers in the hospice.

> *'I went to the house to see this particular lady and I knocked at the door and the next thing the husband opened the door and he had a towel in his hand... and it was just him and the towel in his hand. It had a funny effect on me. It was something about the whole thing of caring and love, here is this man and this big estate and the world out there doesn't know what he is doing and here he is with his towel and washing his dying wife.*' (Pauline, chaplain, par. 106)

Many of the professionals working in palliative care are motivated by wanting to help. One of the nursing staff, Emer, remarked about professionals in health care, 'I think all of us who go into health care have a need to help and to fix. We are "fixer uppers".' Home care seemed to present more challenges for the nurses to 'fix things', as there was a delicate balance between helping and providing a service while respecting the patient and family's ability to manage the situation for themselves.

> *'In home care you sit down and you are a guest in their house, you are seeing what makes them tick, you are only supporting them, you are not taking over from them.*' (Marie, nurse, par. 12)

Home care presented a contrast with the in-patient service of the hospice, where it is possible to care for and observe patients on a 24-hour basis; not being able to do this and accepting that the family can manage without this level of professional observation was sometimes difficult. Lorraine talked about managing her own anxieties and worries about the patient and having to remind herself that the family can cope.

> *'There are some patients that you'll think of at eight o'clock in the evening, and wonder is he OK now, but that's normal, you know. But it's not normal to ring the family and ask, are you OK?*' (Lorraine, nurse, par. 78)

'Empowering' and supporting

According to the professional staff I spoke with in the study, most people have a preference to die at home, and this required considerable support for family members, who may initially have been unaware of the level of support that the dying person needed and the implications of this for the carers.

> '*Very demanding on them, it really is. Some families take it on and don't really know what it is going to be about, some people take it on because it is going to be short-term. But then it turns into a very long term and they are very stressed out and sometimes a little respite in a hospice and then they can go home and do it and do it the way they want, you know. But it is very stressful, especially too if they start running into problems with nausea, agitation, you know, and the person changes and they are not the person that you thought they were. They have their own lives as well, some people have their own families.*' (Marie, nurse, par. 20)

The decision to continue caring for the dying person at home or to go into the hospice was made by the family and the patient. Marie, a home care nurse, talked about supporting the family in whatever decision they came to. This was a two-way process, in which the family were given the information about the likely progression of the illness and what the implications of care would be and the family talked about their own resources and needs.

> '*They can decide what they want to do and at the last minute if they decide they want to come into a hospice then I will do my best to do it. And as long as they are listened to and help them make some sort of sense if they want to do it.*' (Marie, nurse, par. 38)

Moving from home to hospice

Although home care staff supported and facilitated families in caring for the dying person at home, some patients moved to the hospice to die. There were a variety of reasons why this happened.

As the illness progressed, sometimes the physical symptoms became more problematic and the burden of care then became too great; family members became exhausted, particularly if the patient had been dying over an extended period and there were small numbers of family members available to help with the care. While Pauline, one of the chaplains, talked about, in one instance, being struck by the level of intimacy between one man and his dying wife, for some families very intimate care was difficult to give, and for some patients difficult to accept from family members.

> '*For me to give somebody a bath is nothing, it's second nature to do that. But to ask maybe a wife or a daughter or maybe a son to do that for a parent or a spouse or whatever, that is not natural for them and the patient themselves, parents don't feel comfortable, say, with a family member giving them a bath. This is a private thing*.' (Emer, nurse, par. 44)

Sometimes the dying person and/or the family initiated the move into the in-patient unit because of a belief that physically dying at home would cause problems for family members.

> '*People have decided not to die at home. And some of the reasons that people have is because of the stress that it would cause their greater family. We have had certainly people who have died here because their relatives have stated that they wouldn't be able to sleep in the bed again if they died in the bed. They would be aware of the distress their death would cause somebody.*' (Margaret, doctor, par. 77)

While patients had the opportunity, in theory, to avail of social work or chaplaincy support at home, sometimes this wasn't possible because either the resources of the service were unavailable at the time requested or it was difficult for patients to avail of these services as family members may have resisted these interventions, particularly that of social work. The interwoven relationship between the patient and family meant that it could be difficult for the patient to say what they needed without upsetting the family. A move to the hospice provided some dying patients with an opportunity to talk about their own distress to someone outside the family and to receive spiritual and psychological support for themselves.

> '*I have had one or two people say that they want to come here for the spiritual support that would be here. Because the other difficulty that people have sometimes is that the people they are least likely to talk to about all the psychological distress are the people closest to them. For many reasons, they have to be strong for them, to protect them and it is hard to talk, so people find the care here valuable because they can talk to people.*' (Margaret, doctor, par. 87)

In between: the day care service

The day care service at St Theresa's provided clinical, psychological, social and spiritual care for patients as well as being a link for and between community health care professionals, hospice home care teams, the in-patient unit, general hospital and the patients' general practitioner. The purpose of the service was to support patients in staying at home for as long as possible and at the same time to provide clinical and social services, with a weekly assessment of patients. The day care service involved a complex balancing act between the needs of the patients, staff and the service.

Balancing aims

The service aimed to provide clinical assessment and support for patients who were still at home. There was a considerable amount of social activity for patients and the assessment of patients happened in an informal way.

> '*You have to get through talking to all the patients so you suss out all their symptoms and you are aware of any problems that may arise that they might not be aware of, like you are doing a full assessment but it is an informal full assessment.*' (Geraldine, nurse, par. 38)

The assessment took place during the day-to-day social activities, and from talking to the day care nurses, Geraldine and Catherine, it was clear that they were engaged in constant observation of the patients in day care.

> '*Because we dish out meals and things like that, you end up doing a lot of the practical things. But even just looking around the room you pick up an awful lot and just how they are interacting, are they interacting as much as they were the previous week or maybe they are falling asleep, things like that, you know, you are watching the room continuously.*' (Geraldine, nurse, par. 42)

While assessment was part of the aims of day care, patients had a different set of expectations when they came into the hospice for the day and a balance between these two aspects was sometimes hard to achieve.

> '*It can be difficult because on the one hand, my aim is to find out what exactly is going on with them but their aim is to switch off and not think about what is going on. So you have to balance it and sometimes you don't get to fully assess someone, which is difficult because that is what I am supposed to do.*' (Geraldine, nurse, par. 40)

Incorporated into the day care service were other aspects of care, such as spiritual care. Day care patients could avail of the religious service held daily in the hospice and the chaplain also visited on a daily basis, although the contact with patients was generally informal.

> '*I don't get huge amounts of referrals on paper. What I do is go over and go to the multi-disciplinary team meeting there, which is held every Tuesday morning, and I pick up from that if there are people who might benefit from meeting me or I just go over and just be around, introduce myself and maybe sit for a little while with people. And then some people, you know that they need you and you just stay with them or some people just want to talk about the weather, that's fine too.*' (Bernadette, chaplain, par. 60).

Balancing support

The day care service was nurse-led and coordinated care with health care services in the community and the patient's doctor, outside of St Theresa's. Both Catherine and Geraldine worried about getting the balance right between a social service and a medical one. As the aims of day care included social contact and support and maintaining people at home within their own medical support systems, Geraldine felt that the presence of a full-time medical service in day care, while it may have been beneficial for providing swift symptom recognition and control, would focus too much on the physical symptoms and bring patients into the full service before they needed this level of intervention and care.

> '*If we had a doctor down here full-time in one way it would be great because you could have symptoms recognised straight away but in another regard you would pull them too much into the service too soon. You are trying to get that balance right, it is all contradictory but it is trying to get a balance. They feel they are part of a service and they are getting what they want from the service but yet you are trying to facilitate them staying at home in their own normal support services and their local GP for as long as possible.*' (Geraldine, nurse, par. 44)

Catherine talked about achieving a balance between the social activities and looking after people medically, but felt that the activities were of no use if patients' symptoms were not looked after.

> '*Maybe this is because I'm coming from a nursing background but if they come in with symptoms all the lovely things in the world won't help if they go home with the same symptoms .... It's trying not to make it too medicalised so it is not turned into mini outpatients it's trying to keep the balance and meet needs at the same time.*' (Catherine, nurse, par. 129)

Balancing resources

The day care service, in providing weekly assessments of patients, was considered by staff to alleviate the workload of the home care team, although the home care services were still working with some patients and families. Day care was also considered as respite for full-time carers at home.

> '*It is symptom management for the patient, so that symptoms that you need to check up can get checked on a weekly basis; so that you won't need the home care nurses to call in so much. It is for respite for the family because you know the way illness can frustrate the family and it is respite for the family away from the patient.*' (Geraldine, nurse, par. 50)

For patients who did not have family members to care for them or were socially isolated in some way, a once-weekly visit may not have been enough to provide the social contact that would have been of benefit to them, and the staff I spoke with found it difficult to balance the needs of patients with those of the resources available.

> '*There are a lot of people that are socially isolated that could come four days a week. But then if you are looking at a purely specialist palliative day care service, a lot of those people don't need that, they're lonely, they've no one to make a meal for them, they're frightened, they're anxious, there is a whole lot of reasons. That is the difficulty I find in that, like you are the specialist palliative day care which is great and that is very much the head saying, well, yes, these are the criteria we need. Then the heart, when some little old lady that needs to be here and there's no one at home and hasn't had a bath and all these things. And it's trying to find a balance.*' (Catherine, nurse, par. 149)

A stepping-stone

The day care service was seen, by the day care staff, as an introduction to St Theresa's. Acting as a stepping-stone for a possible admission to full-time care in the in-patient unit in the future, patients were considered, by staff, to become more familiar and comfortable with the place and the staff. Some of the patients who attended day care were perceived as having social needs, such as a lack of social support at home. These needs may make it more likely that the patient would be admitted to the in-patient unit as the illness progressed. If the experience of day care was positive for patients, it was felt by staff to influence favourably their perception of the in-patient unit and allay fears concerning admission to the hospice.

> '*It is also an introduction as well, if people have come to day care and perceived it as a positive experience for them then they are often much more open to the idea of coming in if they were fearful about the idea of a hospice. Most people view a hospice as the place where you come in, at the very final stages of illness, to die.*' (Carol, doctor, par. 88)

The day care service was an introduction to the hospice building and the people who work there; however, this was an introduction for the patient only and the contact with the family was limited. Both the day care nurses felt that this was often unsatisfactory as they had an incomplete picture of the patient and what was happening in the home that might affect the patient.

> '*We're sort of the stepping-stone or the introduction to in-patients. ... the one drawback to day care is that we do not get to meet the family. You're talking to people over the phone and you're trying to assess things over the phone and it is difficult.*' (Catherine, nurse, par. 163)

When day care staff became aware of difficulties within the family they often alerted the home care services. It was clear that the degree of contact between the day care service and the family increased as the patient's physical condition worsened and if there were health problems with the patient that could lead to an admission to the in-patient service. The closer the likelihood of admission to the hospice in-patient unit became, the more contact professional staff had with the family. At the same time, as the physical condition of the patient worsened, families also contacted the day care nurses and other professionals concerning admission more frequently.

> '*We have one gentlemen, he is unwell but could hold on until the next week but his wife is very stressed out and when you ring her on the phone she says "I'm not talking, you'll only upset me" and the phone goes down, so the home care go down to see her and to offer support for her. So that's the one drawback to day care, you don't see where the person lives, their circumstances or the family. But often we would invite the families to come in, maybe on their first day. Just to meet them and see how things are so that they know a face and a name when you ring up. We would usually, when somebody is ill, if there was something we were worried about, ring the family and just check in just to say hello, how are things, how's it going, you know just to support, they know someone's there on the phone. Sometimes they take it up when they have an issue, when there is a problem, when they are worried. Often it would be to come in as things start to deteriorate, about future plans, what's the chances of coming in, what can we do, we would try and have family meetings you know when issues come up.*' (Catherine, nurse, par. 178)

A place apart: the in-patient unit

The in-patient unit provided an opportunity for staff to develop a relationship with the patient and the family in a setting in which the patient, rather than the palliative care professionals, was the visitor. Having the opportunity to get to know the patient and the family and their particular likes and dislikes was viewed by the nursing staff in the in-patient unit as enhancing the care of the patient.

> '*It is nice if you have the time beforehand to get to know them, to know their likes and dislikes and what their family want. A good death too for somebody is not just doing what they want to do, it is if the family are happy and that is what I would consider a peaceful death, it is when everybody, all their expectations are, you know.*' (Marie, nurse, par. 24)

Changing roles

In the in-patient unit, in a general sense, family ceased to be the main carers, although Helen, whose husband had died at St Theresa's, was 'allowed' to continue the daily care of her husband in the in-patient unit. This may have been a result of the caring role that Helen had engaged in for a long period before her husband was admitted to the in-patient unit.

> '*I still needed to feel that I was the main carer and I was doing what I could for him but it just wasn't possible for the last two months. So I talked about that here and they allowed me to still do what I was doing at home only it was in this kind of environment where the medical or the nursing support was here.*' (Helen, administration and family member, par. 17)

Members of the home care team switch from being a visitor in the patient's home to being a visitor in the in-patient unit, and Peter, a home care doctor, talked about the team in the in-patients unit 'taking over totally' the care of patients that had previously been looked after at home.

> '*I'm only a visitor as well. And it is nearly more for me than for them, it's better if the team down there takes over totally unless for some very special reason, which there can be sometimes, people want to see you but the ongoing emotional and spiritual care does pass to that team and it's probably better there. The people who come in are weak and they are within their last days alive, I don't want them spending their last energies on me because they knew me before. They need to talk to the team who is looking after them because they have to know how things are there and they need energies for their own families and friends.*' (Peter, doctor, par. 81)

When I spoke to some of the home care nurses informally about this issue, however, they felt it depended on the circumstances. Sometimes a home care nurse was familiar with complex family issues and then might attend a family meeting. If they had a more personal relationship with the patient it was not unusual to visit the patient, although they would not be involved in the nursing care.

For some family members, lifting the burden of care by admitting the dying person to the in-patient service restored aspects of the previous relationship.

> *'It gave me a chance because I had fallen into the role of carer for so long the actual relationship, our relationship as a couple had changed so much. And I felt that I had lost that, I was conscious that I wanted to get something back before he died, you know I needed to get that sense of togetherness again. So that, it enabled me to do that here and I had the time and energy because at least I could go home and have a full night's sleep. And come in the morning and spend the whole day here if I wished, which I did.'* (Helen, administration and family member, par. 17)

Hospice as home

Although most people expressed a preference for staying at home, sometimes the move into a specialist setting became necessary, and considerable emphasis was placed on creating a pleasing and home-like environment.

> *'You want people to feel as at home as they can because I suppose the whole day care and home care ethos is to keep patients at home for as long as possible. So when patients come in here they haven't managed to stay at home so you want them to feel as much at home here.'* (Geraldine, nurse, par. 202)

There was clearly an intention to create a home-like atmosphere in the hospice, as described in Chapter 5. Part of that atmosphere was familiarity with some staff; owing in part to the small size of St Theresa's, it was easy to meet and engage with members of staff, especially if they were involved in administration and working at the reception.

> *'To me it's like a little home, you know, like you might go into a big major hospital and you will get a hello from a few nurses, especially if someone is in there for a long time, but everybody here knows everybody.'* (Monica, administration, par. 221)

A further aspect of this deliberate policy to create a home-like atmosphere in the hospice was the emphasis on home cooking in the canteen, which was part of the contract requirements for the caterers.

> *'That was the objective from day one, it was home cooking; it was never going to be a flash restaurant because that wasn't what was required here.'* (Carmel, kitchen staff, par. 159)

As already described, Sr Bridget's philosophy of providing the 'best of everything' guided the decoration and furnishing of the hospice. This raised a question as to whether the hospice was too beautiful, particularly for patients and family members whose own home surroundings may have contrasted considerably with this.

> *'I think it is beautiful but it is comfortable and it is homely rather than it is too good to be in it and you are afraid of touching things and I think that is important. If you are having somebody comfortable the environment, yes it is nice that it looks nice but it shouldn't be so nice that you are afraid to touch.'* (Sheila, doctor, par. 106)

Some patients, however, did find the hospice too much of a contrast with their own surroundings at home and needed to return to their own environment.

> *'One man, when he realised he was not going to get better and we were not going to make him better, he wanted to go home immediately. So he went home that evening, it had to be, we had to use a wheelchair, we had to get a volunteer driver in to get the mini bus and he had to be carried up three flights of stairs to his flat, with drug addicts and pushers at every turn. But that was where he wanted to be. He wanted to be at home there in his own world.'* (Sheila, doctor, par. 96)

A controlled space

Although St Theresa's tried to create a home-like atmosphere, the hospice was not home, and Noirin, a nurse who had worked both in home care and the in-patient unit, found it difficult to see patients sitting in their pyjamas or nightclothes during the day, and felt that it was easy to forget that a patient had a life outside. Her experience of knowing people in their own home had provided a clearer boundary between the nurse and the patient and the family.

> '*I think people tend to come to a unit or a hospital as such, and they're sitting in the bed in their pyjamas and you know at home they are really their own person and again it depends on the personality of the patient, some people are quite happy to be here and be away from the family home but I used to see it visiting people at home where I was a guest in their house, it would mean that there would be boundaries that you would be aware of whereas here sometimes you forget that this person actually had a life outside of these four walls.*' (Noirin, nurse, par. 48)

Noirin talked about the in-patient unit in terms that contrasted with the view of it as a cosy home-like place.

> '*It definitely turns the table around because this is our territory and we know how things run and in a sense you know we take things away from people, like all of a sudden they are in their pyjamas all day, which they will not be at home. We take their tablets away and we give them tablets when we think it is the right time to give them tablets.*' (Noirin, nurse, par. 52)

Nevertheless, the level of control that was exercised with patients, family and visitors was, on occasion, beneficial for patients as it allowed them space and respite from family attention and constant visitors.

> '*But then it can be great, the respite here is brilliant and a few patients have said they found it really good, just to get a break from, you know, people at home might be fussing over them and visitors all the time, they are not able for it so they come in here. At least then we can actually say, "Look, he's really tired, maybe come back tomorrow"; we can actually have some control on it, whereas they might feel at home they can't control it at all.*' (Noirin, nurse, par. 56)

The in-patient unit provided space and time away from family and visitors for the patient but also provided space and respite for family members. Helen, whose husband died in the hospice, felt that lifting the total burden of care from her helped her regain something of the relationship between herself and her husband before he died, and Noirin also talked about a woman who seemed transformed after her husband was admitted to the hospice.

> '*I saw a woman transform within two days. Her husband was in and she was looking terrible and then I saw her two days later and she had the make-up on and she just looked like a completely different person, just purely, a bit of space and a couple of nights' sleep.*' (Noirin, nurse, par. 62)

Creating a peaceful atmosphere

A peaceful environment for the patient and family members seemed to promote reflection and acceptance of what was happening. The atmosphere created in the hospice was described as peaceful and tranquil by many of the people working there; Maeve, one of the volunteers, described it as 'like stepping into a slow stream'.

There was a sense in the hospice that the physical setting was a place apart, and this sense of being apart from the outside world was seen as supportive for some patients.

> '*I often see the hospice as a place, a kind of stepping aside for somebody, to take stock of what is going on. I have seen people come in here sometimes, restless and worried because they are in their terminal stage of cancer. They come in agitated and after a couple of days or weeks here somehow there seems to be this peace that comes and I wonder sometimes if it is something to do with stepping aside from the business of out there.*' (Bernadette, chaplain, par. 170)

Having the opportunity to talk to staff, in particular chaplains, about the process of dying and their fears and worries about this may be one of the reasons why people decide to come into the hospice to die. It may be that, while families can provide huge support, there was a pressure on the patient to be brave and not show their fear or vulnerability. The hospice was a safe place for some patients to acknowledge their impending death and to express their fears.

> *'Sometimes out there it can be "You will be grand, just give yourself another few days, another few weeks or whatever" and everybody knows that is not the truth. When they come in here that is not being said to them ... It gives them a chance to maybe feel what is going on and be allowed to express it. Whereas often out there, they can't do that because people don't want to hear it.'* (Bernadette, chaplain, par. 172)

The presence of death

One of the aspects of being in the in-patient unit in the hospice was that death was always around, and this necessitated acknowledging that death was imminent.

> *'One of the things that sometimes comes up, you know, with families not wanting to tell patients that they have cancer. And we say when they come here, they are going to see people dying all around them. You can't pretend that you are in a hospital.'* (Jean, administration, par. 140)

For some patients the presence of other dying people helped in coming to terms with a terminal illness; however, multi-bed rooms for patients, rather than single rooms, also created difficult situations.

> *'It is very difficult when you have an anxious situation in a four-bedded room, it is having a huge knock-on effect with everyone else.'* (Geraldine, nurse, par. 123)

For patients the constancy of the death of patients in the same room was an uncomfortable reminder that death was inevitable and close. For some patients who may have been in the hospice for a few months there was the additional loss of friends they had made.

> *'I think it is too much to have to share with people that are dying. It can be good on one level because sometimes it would help with the realisation with the people that they are dying. But it is very sad ... for patients to see others die ... and for a lot of patients*

> *that have been in for quite a while they would want a list of the patients that they have seen die, list them all and they would probably list them in an order.'* (Geraldine, nurse, par. 214)

Although the proximity of death was hard for some patients, others dealt with this situation with humour.

> *'There was a man, he was a very funny man and people kept dying in the room and he said "This is like being on death row", and a lady who also had people dying in her room said "I'm still alive, I must be standing at the wrong bus stop".'* (Susan, administration, par. 218)

Staff seemed to recognise the impact of this on patients in the four-bedded rooms. It appeared to be a frequent occurrence that patients in the same room died within hours of each other—this happened several times during the course of the study. When resources allowed it, i.e. when there was a single room available, new patients that were not expected to live very long were not admitted to the four-bedded rooms because of the possible impact on the remaining patients in the four-bedded room.

> *'They are conscious that people that are here maybe have seen a lot of death this week, I've heard it said "We are not bringing in [to a four-bedded room] somebody who is going to die today".'* (Jean, administration, par. 146)

Some of the staff also found it difficult when deaths occurred very close together over a short period. The emotional labour of being with and supporting relatives was very difficult for some of the nurses, especially if deaths occurred with little respite.

> *'I remember there was a young nurse there and she was saying what she found really hard was when a whole group died, maybe two or three deaths all together, and again going to the mortuary. And having to cope with having to face people, the relatives' grief, not just once but perhaps two or three times during a weekend, you know.'* (Mary, administration, par. 70)

The hospice setting presented patients and family members with the inevitability of death, and this was also the case for staff, but not all of the staff were comfortable with this. In the preceding chapters, it was clear that some of the nursing staff were attracted to working in palliative care because of the opportunity to focus on caring for patients and because the multi-disciplinary and organisational aspects were also attractive, not because palliative care involved working with patients who were dying. Part of the diploma for palliative care nursing involves an examination of personal thoughts and feelings about death; not all the nurses at St Theresa's had undergone this training. Angela, a nurse in the in-patient unit who had not been trained as a palliative care nurse, enjoyed working in St Theresa's because of the organisational structures and values but did not enjoy working with patients who would not get better.

> '*To my mind you could never be ready for death, you know, but of course I am fully aware of the reason, one of the reasons that it doesn't suit me is because of my own, I haven't worked on mine, my situation, my own death.*' (Angela, nurse, par. 58)

For other staff members, both professionals and others who did not deal directly with patients, the constant presence of dying patients in the hospice led to a frequent confrontation with their own mortality; some aspects such as age seemed to act as triggers for facing this.

> '*I have sat there at admissions and actually looked at the ages and I have thought, I have suddenly looked at what I am doing and realised that I am hoping they are all older than me, they are not. And the day there were more younger than me I felt extremely uncomfortable. I was looking at a list of people younger than me that were not going to get better and you have to see your own death and your own attitude to life.*' (Joan, social worker, par. 52)

While the training for palliative care nurses formally provided a reflection process about death and dying, confronting death on a daily basis seemed to engage some staff in an informal personal process of reflection about death and about the impact of a terminal diagnosis.

> '*When I think I am well but have a limited life-span left then I think of the things I like to do. But when I try to picture what it's like to be told that you are not going to live long I realise that you probably wouldn't dwell on those things. You would dwell on the people who matter to you, what you are going to say to them. What you want them to know, I doubt if many people anguish about what they don't get done but I think they anguish about who they haven't spoken to.*' (Joan, social worker, par. 73)

An unsuitable setting

Not all patients and family members wished to die in a hospice. For some patients, staying in a hospital setting where the focus was on cure rather than death represented hope in some form or other.

Some family members resisted the non-medical aspects of palliative care, since accepting the services of social workers or chaplains involved acknowledging and accepting that death was inevitable, as in their view only doctors could help. This position, although respected by palliative care professionals, was difficult for some staff to accept as it involved witnessing people in distress.

> '*He steadfastly refused to be involved with anyone other than doctors. In fact he used the words "Keep those social workers and counsellors away from me". That's fine and everybody respected that. It is only now that his wife is at death's door and he accepts that there is nothing else, that he has asked for this. It did not come from us and we respected his statement that he did not want it. The nurses were itching to push it a bit, they were finding it hard to see him in great need and his refusal to have extra help but they had to tolerate their discomfort. So now it's totally different, he feels "I can't handle this" but he said "Even three weeks ago I wouldn't have wanted to know you because I didn't want to regard my wife as dying or in need. I was still waiting for a miracle and still refusing to believe this can happen and I didn't want to have any contact with anybody except*

> *doctors because doctors can cure you".*' (Joan, social worker, par. 142)

Peter, one of the home care doctors, talked about the 'entangled web' of ideas about palliative care and how by allowing the palliative care professionals in the door there was a sense that you allowed death in the door. It seemed to be quite similar in the in-patient unit, where some patients seemed to feel that the specialist setting almost caused one to die—because you have entered the hospice you are going to die rather than you are going to die and therefore you go to the hospice.

> '*Some people do not want to come in here because there can be a feeling that you die because you come in here, not that you come here because you are dying. For some people it does help to say "Yes I am dying and therefore I need to come into the hospice". However, because people die here it prevents some people from coming in, some people want to stay in acute hospitals because there is hope even if they know themselves they are dying but they are dying where there is hope.*' (Sheila, doctor, par. 92)

Managing social space and social ties

The in-patient unit is the 'territory' of the professionals, and while it was clear that considerable efforts were made to present a home-like atmosphere, the in-patient unit is an institution and as such the physical and social space was managed by the professionals. The values and aims of the model of care and those of the organisation place a high value on the needs of patients and family members; at the same time there are many patients and family members and there may, at times, be competing or conflicting needs. These aspects were managed by the professional staff, in particular the nursing staff, who are in closest proximity to the patients and family members.

The family

Family was defined by the dying person or a member of the family and included people, apart from blood or marriage relatives, who were important to the dying person. One of the mechanisms for management was to ascertain who was to be informed when the patient died, and this indicated to the staff the order of relationships with the dying person. Sometimes there were the complications of extra-marital relationships which needed to be accommodated, often by bringing in a visitor late at night when the 'real' family was not there.

> '*When patients are admitted here, the person, or whoever the next of kin is, or whoever is supporting them or depending how well they are, they define the family. Who matters to you, who are the important people and occasionally it will be non-family, closest friends, that type of person is included as well. Occasionally it will be a dotted line, now and again we get the complexities of extra-mural, extra-marital relationships and significant others and there are discussions and manipulations and stuff about allowing somebody to visit but not when the real family is there and all that. Sometimes you will have these levels, somebody who is very important to them could be visiting but will be coming very late at night and not to be bumping into everyone else, all of that. But the patient, if possible, or the next of kin or the immediate family who is constantly with [the patient] would give you the names and they list who they would want informed when they die and that's a good guide to matters like that.*' (Joan, social worker, par. 170–6)

The presence of families

Family size in Ireland tends to be large, although this is now changing. Large numbers of family members were often present in the in-patient unit, and while families were observed as being a source of considerable strength and comfort, there were also times when the presence of family members caused problems, mainly because of pre-existing family tensions, a problem exacerbated by family size.

Some of the staff, such as Elizabeth who worked in reception, observed that the physical space in the hospice often became crowded with family members, especially as it was quite usual for extended family to visit frequently. Although staff did remark on this, I never felt, in the time I spent there, that the hospice was unduly crowded or uncomfortable, although there were certainly, from time to time, large numbers of people around.

> '*I often feel sorry for the patient, like you look at some of them and they have swarms of visitors. Maybe they have five children and also brothers and sisters and maybe their children have children and all these people are constantly in all the time. Maybe in the room or in the smoke room or up and down having cups of tea and taking turns sitting in the room.*' (Elizabeth, administration, par. 134)

Christine, one of the nurses in the in-patient unit, felt that with large numbers of visitors it was difficult for patients to get space for themselves.

> '*The patient finds that they can't get space for themselves and there are constant visitors and that might only be family but if there is a big family that they can never get a little bit of space for themselves.*' (Christine, nurse, par. 8)

The final days and hours present specific management problems for the nursing staff. For family members this can be an anxious time, as frequently this was a new and often frightening experience as well as a difficult emotional time. Staff, on the other hand, were familiar with the physical experience of death and aware, from previous experience, of potential difficulties. Some of the anticipated difficulties concerned the behaviour of family members, who might be anxious and tense, and the nursing staff felt that these emotions could be transmitted to patients. When the nursing staff felt that this was the case they often engineered an opportunity to observe the patient without family members being present.

> '*It may be a case where the family's anxiety is making the patient worse, I might say, listen, why don't you slip down and get something to eat and I will sit here and that gives me a chance to really suss out how anxious they are. In some cases, you will find that they relax more when you are there and the family has gone away.*' (Geraldine, nurse, par. 92)

The family were left alone with the patient when death was imminent and for a short while after the death. Some of the nursing staff encouraged the family to say a few last words to the dying person.

> '*I always say don't be frightened, take a little bit of time, say the things you'd like to say and I would give them time immediately, say, after the death. I would leave them so that they can have their own chat around the bed, spend a little bit of time without my presence there and go back in then.*' (Deirdre, nurse, par. 150)

> '*We would always take time, step back and leave the family as much time as they wanted around the bed, whatever they wanted.*' (Christine, nurse, par. 132)

The short- and long-term welfare of family members was considered part of the care in the final days and hours before death. The nurses that I spoke with considered that it was important for the family to be present at the death as this helped the family afterward; however, managing both the physical presence of the family in the hospice and the welfare of family members over a long period placed strain on the nursing staff.

> '*We would do our utmost to have family with them. When you look at the patient, if you feel that they're low or that you think that there is a possibility of them dying, we would say for some of the family to stay. You might have them staying for, we had one lady and the family was staying for a week literally, I mean, she'd be down, you'd think she was going to die and then she'd rally round again. Very difficult on the family, so you're trying to avoid that situation as well, that they're not there for the long haul. I think that probably it makes the bereavement a little bit better if they're there when the patient actually dies, so we would try our utmost to have the family there.*' (Deirdre, nurse, par. 69)

A continuing relationship

Relationships continued after death with the person who has died, the family and the palliative care services. The relationship with the family continued with follow-up calls to family members after a two-week interval as part of the bereavement services provided by St Theresa's. Family members continued to have a relationship with the deceased, although this was manifested in a variety of ways.

The family and the hospice

Some family members continued to connect with the in-patient unit for some time after the death. Although there were bereavement follow-up services, sometimes the connection with the hospice took the form of families returning for regular religious services within the unit. Having a Mass said for the deceased is a common practice within Catholicism and this may happen in a parish church, but some families continued their connection with the hospice and returned for Mass there.

> '*Families come back and have a Mass said for the person who died here. People come in and somebody has died and maybe for six months afterwards they will come regularly to Mass here and then it will begin to taper off. Now they can cope and they don't need a crutch anymore.*' (Elizabeth, administration, par. 128)

The family and the deceased

Some family members talked about a continued relationship with the deceased which took different forms and manifested itself in a variety of ways.

The relationship may be internalised on a continuous basis in the lives of surviving family members, and Helen said that she felt her relationship with her husband continued after his death.

> '*He is not in my past, I will never leave him behind, because he is part of me, so in order to move on I have brought him with me. You know, he is part of my present and part of my future because he is part of me... It would be parallel to your life all the time and it crosses your path at times for various reasons, you know. Even on a daily basis.*' (Helen, family member and administration, par. 25–7)

Monica perceived the presence of her deceased mother through physical sensations.

> '*I tell you what and you will think I am mad when I say this. But there are times in my own house and I would get this smell and I would say that's Mam because she used to smoke years ago. There wasn't a smoke smell, I don't know what kind of smell it was but you would get it when you were close to her. I had that for ages afterwards. On the bed, going to bed at night time I would feel her.*' (Monica, family member and administration, par. 129)

The deceased may be a constant presence and a source of help for the family members, and understood in appropriate terms for each family member.

> '*His wife was saying to me last week that they will say out openly in school that Daddy has gone to Heaven and he won't be coming back but one of her daughters says "He has a magic chair beside me and he is always there helping me".*' (Elizabeth, administration, par. 312)

The deceased may also feature strongly in dreams, and Elizabeth, who had suffered depression after the death of her aunt and her mother, felt that this dream resolved the depression.

> '*I had this dream. Someone was calling my name and I sat up and opened my eyes to see who was calling me and it was my aunt and she said "Look at us". And I was looking out over a golden field of corn and there were six beautiful golden girls walking towards me, my mother, all of them, all my mother's sisters and herself. And that was the end of my depression because I felt they had all made it.*' (Elizabeth, family member and administration, par. 312)

Summary

The way in which the location of care shaped and influenced the relationships between patients, families and palliative care professionals is explored in this chapter. It is clear that the patient and the family remained more in control of the level of intervention of the palliative care services when the patient was at home and the palliative care professionals remained as visitors in this setting. However, this position and the dominance of the family culture and values, especially concerning communication and open awareness about issues around death and dying, were sometimes problematic for the palliative care professionals.

In contrast, in the in-patient unit the family members and the patients were visitors and needed to adapt to that location; those unable to do so chose to return home or to remain in hospital. This adaptation involved confronting the inevitability of death in ways that conformed to the organisational values. A deeper engagement with the hospice and palliative care professionals, especially nursing and chaplaincy staff, was facilitated in the in-patient unit, and to a lesser extent in the day care service. Given the emphasis on psychosocial and spiritual aspects of care that was apparent in St Theresa's, this deeper engagement with the palliative care professionals in the hospice focused attention on the spiritual care of patients and families, and this aspect will be explored in the following chapter.

CHAPTER 7
Religion and spirituality

Introduction

The debate in the literature concerning spiritual care and definitions of spiritual care reflects the overlap between religion and spirituality, as discussed in Chapter 2. Religious beliefs and practices can be considered spiritual, but as spirituality is often individually defined, not everyone who considers themselves spiritual engages in religious practice or holds religious beliefs. While these overlaps are not in themselves problematic, they may become so within palliative care as spiritual care is one aspect of the multi-dimensional care provided. If spirituality is individualistic, how can this be known and how can people be cared for spiritually?

The palliative care literature in the past, particularly between 1987 and 1999, reflects a preoccupation with defining spirituality and spiritual care, but little attention has been paid to religious practice and belief, suggesting that these are unproblematic. Religious beliefs and practices have been and still are an important part of everyday life in Ireland, however, and they are not necessarily straightforward or unproblematic. Some of the difficulties arise directly as a result of the role of the Catholic Church in Ireland; others reflect more universal fears and anxieties at the end of life when religious beliefs may not always be helpful.

There was a strong Catholic presence at St Theresa's and an emphasis on spiritual care as part of the care at the hospice. This chapter explores a variety of views, drawn from those I spoke with in the hospice, concerning religious beliefs and practice and their place at the end of life; in addition, it explores their definitions of spirituality and spiritual care.

Religion in Ireland

As outlined earlier, the Catholic Church has had a unique role in the development of Irish society from the middle of the nineteenth century. Religious orders have been intensely involved in the delivery of education and health care, and religion and religious practice are therefore embedded in social practice in Ireland in a way that is not the case certainly in the UK or even in other European Catholic countries such as Italy and Spain. One of the participants in the study remarked that 'you are living in a culture where religion is a very natural thing, because religion is very much a natural part of Irish culture' (Christine, nurse, par. 84). This 'naturalism' of religion in Ireland, however, can be considered as largely a result of the monocultural nature of Irish society and the embedded position of Church organisations in every aspect of Irish society.

Sheila talked about how some patients with no professed religious beliefs will generally, by the time they die, have planned the funeral with the priest and have become incorporated into the cultural way in which death is organised in Ireland. While it could be considered that returning to the Church and religious rituals at the end of life is a way of 'hedging one's bets', it is considerably easier socially, especially for those left behind, to engage with the predominant rituals around death and dying in Ireland, especially as these seem to be a 'natural' part of life in Ireland.

> '*This is what is interesting about being Irish and cultural things changing. We have a number of people here who are brought up Catholics but are not practising; do not want to see clergy. But most of them usually by the time they die here, they will have the priest planning the funeral Mass and all that. It's like it comes back and I think also the culture in Ireland is such that even though you may have people in Ireland who are not church-goers it's like this is the only game in town. When you come to a time when you need something more, what the more is in Ireland is Catholicism and all that goes with it. Church-going, prayers, the sacraments, the works.*' (Sheila, doctor, par. 129)

A tradition of religion

Traditional religious practice was still very important to many of those cared for by the hospice. This was particularly so given the age profile of patients, although religious practice was also important to younger people. The presence of nuns and priests seemed to be reassuring to patients and family members, according to some of the nurses that I spoke with, and Geraldine, in the day care service, felt that some of the day care patients who were unable to attend Mass in their own parish because of lack of mobility welcomed the opportunity to attend Mass on the day they came to the hospice.

Although there was an expectation that older people have a stronger religious adherence, and many did, younger people also demonstrated religious belief and drew strength from it at the time of illness.

> *'We would expect older people to have faith, quite a number of younger people that we meet have huge faith. It may be less conventional, and then a lot of people turn to religion in a sense of, trying to get an answer to their needs. For some, it would be deep, I am just thinking of one couple, in their thirties.'* (Peter, doctor, par. 146)

Changing religion

While Ireland is still predominantly Catholic, the nature of religious beliefs has changed somewhat. The view of God as a judgemental figure is very much a pre-Vatican II (1963) one. Many patients and family members were raised with this concept of a judgemental God and a sense of obligation toward strict religious adherence. Some older members of the staff reflected this tradition and the central importance of the sacraments and prayer.

> *'I would be saying if I was a visitor or if I was a family member and I was coming in to see my dad or my mother and Mass was on would I not just stop off for the Mass or bring them up to the Mass? Whereas I might be down there at Mass on a Sunday if I am working and you would see the family members going by and going in to the room and bringing the person out for a walk. I would know that RC was on their form but obviously it isn't important, that was just something that was there when they were born and when they went to school and got the sacraments. And I*

> *don't mean it as a criticism of them, but I think at this stage the religious aspect would be huge.*' (Elizabeth, administration, par. 76)

This view, however, did not necessarily match those of the chaplains at the hospice; Bernadette's view reflected a more modern approach.

> '*I would never say of somebody who hadn't been practising, that person is lost or something, I have often said to the relatives, you know, God doesn't think or behave or act as we do. We have a loving God here, who cares much much more for that person in the bed than any of us, regardless of how much we love this person.*' (Bernadette, chaplain, par. 161)

The comfort of religion

Religion can be a comfort, and particularly so at the end of life. One patient remarked to staff, 'How can you do this dying without a God?' (Margaret, doctor, par. 69). Others found comfort and strength in a sense of something or someone other and larger than themselves.

> '*I feel if they have a connection somehow it gives them a little bit of strength because you know they are depending on another power, another person, maybe to help them through a situation.*' (Bernadette, chaplain, par. 70)

For some people the familiar rituals of prayers and the sacraments provided reassurance and comfort.

> '*I suppose people are trying to make some sense of this and what does it all mean. A man I saw yesterday was trying to make sense of this and he would say he is getting consolation from prayer… Prayer was giving him some help. He said "I probably have done more praying than I have ever done in my life in the last couple of weeks". So you get the sense of, you know, people who live their lives without thinking that much about it but it's part of them and then they call on it.*' (Peter, doctor, par. 21–3)

The Sacrament of the Sick

The Sacrament of the Sick, the anointing with oils, appeared to bring consolation and peace to those who received it. This sacrament was perceived by the chaplains to open up a channel to the power of God, and they often spoke of the availability of this power that can be accessed through this sacrament and a sense of God's presence with the patient at this time. The chaplains also spoke of the opportunity to 'hand things over', and to avail of the power of God, and by doing so removing the necessity of discussion. In a sense, the communication that underpins palliative care was seen by the chaplains as something unseen and unspoken between the patient and God. This was observed not just by the chaplains but also by the nursing staff.

> '*For me observing people who have received the Sacrament of the Sick they feel that they are getting a sense of grace for this sacrament. For some people that they get a lot of inner peace from the sacrament, I have yet to see someone refuse the sacrament, apart from those who want nothing to do with the Church.*' (Christine, nurse, par. 94)

Prayer

Prayers also formed an important part of the comfort that was derived from religious practice. Karen, one of the nurses, observed that 'a lot of people do get a lot of strength from prayer' (Karen, nurse, par. 46). In the in-patient unit at the hospice, prayers were a useful mechanism for providing clues for family (for instance, for indicating the closeness of the moment of death) and gave people, at a difficult and tense moment, something to do. For nursing staff, saying prayers with the family members provided an opportunity for unobtrusive observation of both the patient and the family.

> '*I'd ask the family would you like to say a little prayer, you know the time is near and we'll say a little prayer to give him strength and to see him on his way more or less so. Then we have prayers that we say, they are very gentle prayers or if they would like some,*

> *a decade of the Rosary as the patient is dying or after the patient has died, we would say it. It would be very unobtrusive as well, that the family sort of has time to grieve for, sometimes they would say we'll say a prayer now or whatever, so you sort of judge it at the time and see.*' (Deirdre, nurse, par. 91)

Prayers seemed to be a culturally appropriate way, at the moment of death and shortly afterward, of providing opportunities and openings for communication with the family.

> '*Just for communication, you know, when you've said the prayers you can sort of say something and people will talk back to you then and that is nice, when you're getting a feedback to how they're feeling, or you can ask open questions that'll sort of entice them to talk about how they are feeling.*' (Deirdre, nurse, par. 140)

Some repetitive prayers, such as the Rosary, were perceived as having a meditative quality. One chaplain spoke of asking family members to say a decade of the Rosary after someone has just died. The repetitive nature of the prayers had a soothing effect and it was observed that, while family members may have been distraught initially, by the time the decade of the Rosary was complete most family members were calm.

> '*Like some people, or you know, maybe a decade, you know, ten Hail Mary's and it can be enough just to, because they're at a loss as well as to what to do.*' (Deirdre, nurse, par. 148)

Pilgrimage

Pilgrimage is an important tradition within the Catholic Church, and pilgrimage to Lourdes, in particular, was an important aspect of traditional Irish Catholicism. This tradition, although now less important, is still present, and particularly so with people who are terminally ill. For some patients and family members, a pilgrimage to Lourdes may represent a hope for cure of the terminal illness. This aspiration, when articulated, also provided clues for palliative care professionals about the level of understanding concerning the illness and the closeness of death and the degree to which family members may feel powerless in the face of what is happening.

> '*I remember seeing somebody and he was on his deathbed and the daughter wanted to bring him to Lourdes and I was thinking what are you bringing him to Lourdes for? You are talking about going to Lourdes next September or August. He is not going to be here that long, it is amazing actually how many people would want to go to Lourdes... to feel like she couldn't do anything else.*' (Marie, nurse, par. 83–8)

An interesting aspect of pilgrimage to Lourdes was the change it brought. Patients and family members travelled with an expectation or hope of cure, and while this did not occur the journey and the experience were transformative for family members, perhaps even more so than for the dying person.

> '*It is very important for a considerable percentage of the population we deal with. What does it do? I have puzzled about this, in the hospital and in the hospice. I think some people go there hoping for a cure and that does not happen and there can be a frustration to it. But most people go there hoping to get some solace, some strength to get them through what lies ahead. And in a sense the miracle is getting that strength, getting that solace. A lot of people have come back saying that they have found peace there. For themselves, not the patient who is dying but the family members who have been there with the patient, that they have got peace. They have got some understanding through being there and I think that is the miracle.*' (Kevin, social worker, par. 60)

The problem of religion

While religion can provide great comfort and strength for patients and family members, some aspects of religious belief and practice caused problems.

Guilt

For some people, fear of death was not about the loss of self or the end of life but about facing the repercussions for actions in this life. These concerns were not always articulated and were difficult to establish.

> *'She came in several times for symptom control and they could never make any difference; she had a panicky thing, a constant thing. By doing certain things, by asking things at the right time I found that she felt that she was not going to go to heaven... I came back and gave the feedback, like she didn't say "I don't think I am going to go to heaven" or "I'm going to hell", she said things like "I'm not as good a person as you think I am" or things like that. I said I think she is afraid of the afterlife and people said "No, she is afraid of dying, she is afraid of a terrible death". And I said "I think it is more about a bad conscience but it's just a hunch" and eventually I asked her whether she would like to see a priest. She made a confession and it may not have been a necessary one even in the priest's terms but when I saw her the next day she said, "I don't feel so sick anymore" and she didn't seem to relate it to that but she did say that she made a good confession and it was an enormous relief. And she didn't feel so sick anymore.'* (Joan, social worker, par. 99–107)

Fear

Some people were fearful at the end of life and religious beliefs seemed to be the cause rather than the solution. Other people had a general fear of the unknown and of not knowing what might happen.

> *'We tend to ask about fears or worries and sometimes they can relate them to the mode of dying, the physical things; but probably just as frequently they would be the fear of the unknown, we just don't know what happens after that. It is not necessarily a fear of the things that are not known, it is not knowing for certain what will happen. Sometimes it is fears of very specific things, fears of being judged afterwards, but most often I think it is fear of the unknown.'* (Carol, doctor, par. 126)

For some patients, these fears related very specifically to impending judgement. In the face of death, some people lost the certainty of their religious beliefs, a set of beliefs that had guided and informed the way they had lived.

> '*There are undoubtedly the people who fear what is coming after. Fear about is there a God? Fear, you know, this God that I believed in all my life, well, is he really there now that I am going to find out one way or another, potentially. Or they fear, some of them have a vision of God being unforgiving so they are fearful because twenty years ago, I did x, y and z.*' (Margaret, doctor, par. 41)

A doubting of previously steadfast beliefs was distressing and disturbing for the terminally ill person as it raised very difficult questions concerning the life that had been lived; it also caused considerable distress and difficulty for family members.

> '*He said that he had believed his whole life and now that when he was dying and his death was imminent, he started to wonder, suppose it is not true, suppose there is nothing afterwards, what will happen afterwards? He had a whole fear of the unknown and doubt of his life-long beliefs. His wife was so upset about it, she could not believe that he was experiencing these doubts, and she was saying that it was the devil putting these thoughts in his head, because her beliefs were absolutely unshakeable and she was convinced that it was the devil creating these doubts.*' (Carol, doctor, par. 120–2)

Anger

Many Irish people have had negative experiences with the Catholic Church, and the chaplains, as the representatives of the Church, sometimes bore the brunt of this anger.

> '*This man, he was in a four-bedded room, when he saw the priest, before he came over to him at all, he said "I want nothing to do with that man" and you know he didn't want anything to do with him and he didn't have anything to do with him for his whole time in here. Again, he put it down to, he had had bad experiences along the way and he was going to die his own way, he wasn't going to have anything from the Church.*' (Christine, nurse, par. 84–6)

Problematic beliefs

The nature of religious beliefs was also a particular problem, especially when acceptance of illness had a fatalistic aspect. Interestingly, Bernadette, the chaplain, saw this more traditional view of 'God's will' as being problematic because it missed the opportunity to fully explore or express what was 'going on' for the patient.

> '*I feel that people who have religious beliefs, they do actually support them but sometimes I worry about people, I don't know, can you measure religious beliefs? A person who says it's the will of God and we have to accept this, that troubles me at times. Because my fear for the person who is ill or dying is that they do not get a chance to really express what is really going on for them. The pain remains deep down and they don't want to express this because they have always believed in a religion that says everything is God's will and you accept everything as God's will. … Sometimes when people are restless or in a lot of pain and the doctor's medicine can't control the pain, I wonder, is there what they call spiritual pain or soul pain going on? They are not able to express it because if they express it they are not accepting God's will.*' (Bernadette, chaplain, par. 76–8)

For some dying people, particularly elderly people, God is a judgemental and not necessarily reassuring figure.

> '*So I feel there is a little bit of a struggle there, it depends on how we see God in our lives and the way we actually relate to God, you know. A lot of people were brought up with a God that is standing over us, a judgemental kind of God rather than this beautiful kind of love that is there for us.*' (Bernadette, chaplain, par. 82)

A view of God as judgemental and as a figure of fear also extended to worries and concerns that family members had.

> '*One of the cases where I felt that a family member was really worried, it took that family member quite a while to see that yes, maybe this is the God that loves us all. But actually by the time that the person did die, that family member who would have been*

> *very anxious, had actually settled and was able to say yes, this person, my relative, is okay.*' (Bernadette, chaplain, par. 165)

Spirituality

It is hardly surprising that there have been ongoing debates within the palliative care literature, as discussed in Chapter 1, which have attempted to pin down what spirituality is. In order to provide spiritual care it is necessary to know what spirituality is. A generally accepted definition within the palliative care literature focuses on spirituality as an individual search for meaning. In this research that understanding of spirituality formed only one part of a definition; however, it was clear that spirituality was considered as extremely individualistic.

Definitions of spirituality

The variety of definitions that people held highlighted the difficulty of pinning down this concept and demonstrated the multi-faceted or multi-layered nature of spirituality. Some people that I spoke with understood it as 'what makes you tick, what keeps you going' (Karen, nurse, par. 42), or 'whatever is sacred in people's lives' (Peter, doctor, par. 107), and there was a sense that spirituality was something integral to the individual, right at the core of the person.

A connection

Spirituality in this sense is what is individual about each person and what makes a connection between the individual and the surrounding world, whether or not the surrounding world is understood as encompassing something or someone larger than the individual.

> '*I do believe we are all spiritual people and it is something around "Who am I?", the beauty of life, the beauty of other people, the beauty of nature, the beauty of music, all those different things that touch in to us ... It might not be a God, it might not be a person, but it is something that touches into our whole integrity.*' (Pauline, chaplain, par. 72–4)

This connection, between the individual and the world around, both temporal and spiritual, may be expressed through religious beliefs or a belief in an afterlife, in whatever form that may be.

> '*I think there is a difference between the whole spirituality and the whole religion thing. A definite, a huge difference even though the two can be linked and you know I think we are all spiritual people. We may not all be religious people and I suppose the whole religion thing often is the practice of spirituality that the person is working from, you know, the sacraments, Mass, rituals, the Koran, the Bible, whatever.*' (Pauline, chaplain, par. 72–4)

> '*Some people describe a belief in God but they don't have a formal set of beliefs or they have a belief in an otherness outside of the physical reality.*' (Carol, doctor, par. 108)

Although there was an acceptance of spirituality as being something larger than religious beliefs and practices with an inherent moral code, there was still a sense of 'spiritual' as being understood in these terms.

> '*Whereas before people were very church-orientated, they say their prayers or they were in to the sacraments or whatever. Now there is a lot of people who may not go to church at all and they may not say the formal prayers that we were brought up with, but they are very spiritual people, and very good and very humble.*' (Bernadette, chaplain, par. 62)

For some people, their spirituality or their connection may be centred on relationships; this may be a relationship with God, although religious practice may not form part of that relationship.

> '*For me it is a relationship with my God and a sort of communication, seeing God as part of your life and seeing God as having an effect, an input into it without necessarily every Sunday tripping to the Church.*' (Jean, administration, par. 86)

> *'He was a Catholic and he said to me "I was baptised a Catholic, I will always be a Catholic but I have no desire to receive the sacraments, to see a priest or anything else, I'm fine, God and I have worked things out together, we're fine".'* (Emer, nurse, par. 107)

The connection was also seen as focused on achievements and accomplishments in life, and a sense of values in life, and whether or not they have made a difference.

> *'Spirituality can be made up of a sense of value of life, what has gone before. Did I make a difference or did I have a meaning, where did I fit in?'* (Karen, nurse, par. 48)

There was also an understanding of the extremely individualistic nature of spirituality, although the uniqueness of spirituality caused difficulty; Kevin felt that there often wasn't enough time to do this with each person, especially as patients themselves were not always clear in their own definitions.

> *'You need to address each individual patient's idea of spirituality before you can do anything else in that area and we often don't have that time. Or the patients often may not be that clear themselves, you know. In an Irish context for a lot of the older people that we deal with, I think their spirituality has been very much tied up with their religion and tied up in the Catholic Church. And they haven't separated those concepts out, they have equated spirituality with religion and I think for some people it would be quite different. And for some people their spirituality would not necessarily have as tight a connection with their religion so I think you need to look at what people see themselves.'* (Kevin, social worker, par. 42)

Defining spiritual care

Spirituality was understood as highly individualistic, which suggests that spiritual care itself must be individualistic. Kellehear's model of situational, moral or biographical and religious needs at the end of life provided some kind of framework in spite of the ultimately individualistic nature of spiritual care.

> '*I just know that anything worth knowing about death and dying and what people need, the people that I have been involved with and cared for have taught me. They taught me lessons that I will never learn in a book, no amount of research or anything else. The other thing they taught me was that you can have a definition that sort of gives you a framework from which to work, but most things can't be defined. Because it is so individual, the definition* [of spiritual care] *might fit this person but it won't fit that person, they are all so different.*' (Emer, nurse, par. 131)

When specific needs were identified, these tended to be religious or existential needs rather than situational.

> '*The care would be from the chaplains who would be there every day talking to each patient and talking to their family. To find out, like, not everybody wants, some patients would have a different level of spiritual need; only recently I knew one particular patient and his spiritual needs would have been huge because that is the way he was.*' (Elizabeth, administration, par. 74)

> '*I suppose if I was a patient here what I would be looking for is to talk to somebody about what I might be frightened of, I suppose from the point of view of the spiritual, the afterlife, and just talking through what will happen. I would be quite happy that there is an afterlife and I would be going somewhere but I know I would want the chance to talk to somebody about that, it would be important.*' (Jean, administration, par. 86)

> '*The other thing about spirituality is about meaning of life, that is the purpose of life and death and dying.*' (Sheila, doctor, par. 70)

What emerged about what constitutes spiritual care was a focus on the individual person rather than on categorising different types of need. The emphasis is on 'being there', accompaniment, and on the giving of oneself to another. However, knowing what is appropriate to give and how to 'be there' depended on an existing relationship with the dying person.

> '*It is trying to gauge what they want ... I went in to a lady one day who was on her own. The relative wasn't there for some reason and there was a nurse and a care assistant sitting just by this lady and I just went in and I sat at the other side of the bed. One of the nurses had asked me to go in but I remember sitting there and thinking this is beautiful. You know there were these two people, no relative there, and my feeling was that they were giving her all the comfort and all the things she needed. One was holding her hand and the other person was just rubbing the corner of the bed, and I said this is what it is about really, being there for the person with no fuss.*' (Bernadette, chaplain, par. 153)

> '*For me it is just trying to be with them and accompany them in their struggle.*' (Christine, nurse, par. 34)

> '*It's beginning where the person is, you know, it's sitting there.*' (Pauline, chaplain, par. 78)

Two of the chaplains mentioned to me their unease about the spiritual needs assessment tools that are sometimes used in UK health care settings; they felt that it was not possible to measure spiritual needs and spiritual care in this way. There was also a sense that the very nature of palliative care, i.e. the focus on the patient and the tasks that are inherent in that type of care, was in itself spiritual care because it recognised and respected the person. Respecting the person included not talking about spiritual or religious concerns if it was not appropriate, or meeting religious or spiritual needs no matter how individual they were.

> '*You know, you are going in and you are treating them very well and you are doing everything properly for them and they die very well, they might not talk to you about spiritual care. You might have fed their spiritual care; they might have dealt with that themselves then.*' (Marie, nurse, par. 168)

> '*The whole ethos of hospice, the way I would see it anyway, is that*

> *you are there to accompany the patient and their family. And symptom control would be part of the overall control and that can be for emotional level, physical level, mental level, spiritual level. So I suppose it encompasses the whole spiritual care and spiritual care for me is really accompanying people. You really do walk with the patient and very much the family.*' (Christine, nurse, par. 38)

Spiritual care incorporated all levels of care, including physical care and symptom control. Acknowledging and respecting the individual was considered the essence of spiritual care; accompaniment became the mechanism of meeting needs.

> '*Mostly the only way you can address it is to be aware of it and to create a space that things that are sacred for people are acknowledged and to find out what that is for people.*' (Peter, doctor, par. 144)

> '*To really see what the patient really wants and to try and provide that. And that can only be done if you are really accompanying the patient on a continuous basis, not going in and out but just being with people.*' (Christine, nurse, par. 40–2)

Care offered but not imposed was also seen as a feature of spiritual care, as was accepting and respecting the patients' autonomy and privacy.

> '*If somebody has things that they need to get off their chest, if somebody has difficulty and wants to sort those out and we offer that to them and they know that if you need us, we will be glad to help ... But I don't see the point in stirring things up and getting them more anxious at a point in their lives that they are just devastated on many fronts ... If we have any faith, if you do believe in a God then we say God is all-powerful, all-knowing, all-loving, well if he or she is, then why not leave it up to God...why try to play God?*' (Emer, nurse, par. 121–3)

Summary

It is clear from this study that while religious beliefs and practices such as prayers, pilgrimage and the Sacrament of the Sick were comforting for many patients at the end of life, this was certainly not the case for everyone. The more traditional views of Catholicism, especially those of a judgemental God, gave rise to sometimes problematic beliefs, as did negative past experiences of the Church. The variety of experiences, both negative and positive, highlighted the uniqueness of religious experience in much the same way that spirituality was considered as unique to each person.

Spiritual care was understood as a focus on the individual person, and the emphasis was on 'being there' and accompaniment, but knowing how to 'be there' depended on an existing relationship. The holistic care of patients and families which palliative care aims to give can also be considered to be spiritual care in itself as it focuses on addressing the needs of the person rather than the illness.

The understanding of spirituality which emerged—the uniqueness of the individual and at the same time the connection to whatever is meaningful to the individual—suggests that spirituality is not just about the individual but also about the individual's connection with the social world. The social world is individually constructed and may or may not include a spiritual dimension. The interwoven aspects of the individual and the social are reflected in the understandings of a 'good death' which are explored in the following chapter.

CHAPTER 8
A 'good death'

Introduction

The preceding chapters have explored the complexity of patient-focused care, and it is clear that while this care focuses on the individual there are also relationships with others. Caring for the individual involves a focus on these relationships. The implication of the palliative care model is that the staff, professional and non-professional, and the organisational structures that facilitate this care, as well as those who matter to the dying person, are interwoven through these relationships, to a greater or lesser extent.

This chapter explores the relationship between the dying person, the family and the hospice. Facilitating a 'good death' is a central aim of palliative care, and although a 'good death' is as much about the dying process that may have extended over a considerable time, the final days and hours are the culmination of the relationships in their present form. The primary focus of care is the patient, but there are other needs, such as those of the family, the staff and the organisation. These needs may converge or conflict. The tensions between potentially competing needs are even more evident close to death.

Exploring the concept of a 'good death', therefore, is not simple. There are some general characteristics that seemed to be an important part of a 'good death', certainly from a professional perspective. Resolution, acceptance and peace seemed central to achieving a 'good death', but what these aspects mean and how they are facilitated can be very different for each individual and each family. Death is simultaneously an individual experience and a social experience, and it can be difficult to attain a balance in this duality—retaining the understanding that it is individual while, at the same time, accepting that the experience also belongs to and influences other people.

This chapter explores different aspects of a 'good death'. Firstly, there is an exploration of the characteristics of a 'good death'. Resolution, acceptance and peace emerged in this study as part of a 'good death', although the means of attaining these states can differ. Secondly, the uniqueness of each death and how this uniqueness is accommodated is explored. Thirdly, there will be an examination of how a 'good death' is shaped by the perceptions of family members and staff; and finally an exploration of a 'good death' as one that is in harmony with the beliefs and values of the individual, the family and the organisation and with a natural cycle of life and death.

The culmination of a process

A distinction needs to be made between the process of dying and the final days or hours. The process of dying can be considered as being the period of time from receiving a terminal diagnosis up to the final days and hours. The final days and hours are the culmination of this process of dying. Generally, when participants talked about a 'good death', both these aspects were intermingled. The components of a 'good death' such as peace and acceptance are states attained—or not, as the case may be—during the process of dying.

> *'If people arrive in the terminal stages having put off the thought of death and dying and have tried to remain positive I think there is an awful lot that can still be done in that final stage, to try and make things as good as possible, but it can be more difficult. Dying is a process; I think if people are more open along the way, about what is happening, by and large, I think it lends itself to better deaths.'* (Carol, doctor, par. 48)

Opportunity

Palliative care services are, with some minor exceptions, services for cancer patients, certainly in Ireland. The focus on this patient group meant that services were geared toward patients for whom the prognosis and illness trajectory were known in general terms. This predictability presented the dying process as 'an opportunity' for patients and family members.

> '*Most people die when they are very old and sick and have heart attacks or an accident; you know this is kind of a privilege anyway. If people get this privilege, of knowing they are going to die and are aware enough to think it through, most of them use the time to look at what they really have done in their lives. A few weeks after saying "Oh my God I haven't done", the same people are saying "I have had a good life, I have done a lot in my life, I've had an amazing life"*.' (Joan, social worker, par. 61)

> '*One man whose wife died on Friday last was actually saying this morning that if she hadn't been ill, he would never have taken time off from work and they would never have developed the relationship they developed because they were in each other's company twenty-four hours a day for the last year or so. And it brought their relationship to a new level. Now there are positives and negatives in that. This is a man who is freshly bereaved but I think there is that element there for people and that is both from the patient's point of view and the family point of view.*' (Kevin, social worker, par. 52)

Jean, whose father had died suddenly, echoed this view. While understanding that the knowledge of impending death brought other difficulties, such as coping with anticipatory grief and being able to say goodbye, the opportunity to talk about this and to be with someone was seen as an opportunity.

> '*If my Dad had cancer and was dying for a year, I would have had a chance to say an awful lot of stuff to him. I would have had a chance to be with him in it. So I think that sudden death, I suppose for a long time you are in shock after it because really you were just plodding along in your day-to-day life and then somebody is gone and your whole world changes. ... But I do think there is some benefit to having the time, to have the opportunity to say things, I know you are into a different scenario, how do you say "Goodbye" and how do you cope. I know it would be very hard to be with that and to know he was going to go. But you know, I think I would probably opt for that if I had a choice.*' (Jean, administration, par. 47–50)

Contrasting pictures

Laura, one of the nursing staff in the in-patient unit, described an ideal scenario of a 'good death' that seemed to encapsulate the different components and perspectives very neatly and provides the basis from which to extrapolate the various elements involved.

> '*My ideal would be to admit a patient who knew they were going to die and that a patient would be here long enough to appreciate the facilities. To have a little bit of tender loving care, because a lot of the patients that we get have never had that, and it is nice to be able to give, and it is nice for us, for staff as well, for job satisfaction, to get to know people and get to know their families a little bit. So ideally I would like it for them to be here for a few weeks so you can build up the rapport with them and their family so when the time of death comes that you have some relationship with the patient and the family, it makes it so much nicer for everybody. And then for them to have time as well if there are issues or things that are not resolved, that they have, over those days and weeks, time and support to look at those. If there is unfinished business or letters they would like to write, or wills, to have the opportunity to do that. Their physical symptoms would be controlled and they would be peaceful, the patient would get weaker and drowsier, I would like it if that period was long enough for the family to have that bit of time but not days and days, waiting for somebody to go, which you do see as well. Just a short period of unconsciousness and then the patient would just drift off.... It does happen, some people do have that.*' (Laura, nurse, par. 68–72)

Pauline, one of the chaplains, described a difficult and upsetting death that provided a stark contrast to Laura's ideal death.

> *'He would have known that I was there for him in his dying but he kept looking for a cure and a cure never came, he kept hoping and hoping and hoping and it didn't come. The day he died, I will never forget it. I spent the whole day nearly in the room with him and he was just so frightened at the end. He went from being frightened to being okay, being frightened to being okay, he would have gone*

> *in and out of all those different emotions. He did not want to lie down, because he thought when he lay down, he would die. He kept getting up, getting up and getting up and getting out of bed and he would say "Now please take me out of this bed" and I would say "Look, I can't get you out of bed, you can't stand, you'll fall, I can't take you out of the bed". He was really angry with me then for not getting him out, he was amazing. He was at the sheets, he was at everything and at one stage during the day I had to give him a pillow and he would scream into the pillow and say "I want to scream and scream". And I gave him a pillow and I said "Now scream into the pillow" and he put it up to his face and screamed into the pillow. That was going on and on and all the staff were in that day but we couldn't get him to settle, he didn't sleep. He was terrified of death. He asked me to get him tea and biscuits, and I got him tea and biscuits, and later on in the day he asked me for soup. He felt that by not lying down he was not going to die, by eating he was going to live. There was a whole lot of things and people in and out, nurses, doctors, everybody ... eventually he kind of spun, he kind of wore himself down and died the next day. But I was very upset by his death.'* (Pauline, chaplain, par. 35–7)

Aspects of a 'good death'

Resolution, acceptance and peace emerged in this study as three core aspects of a 'good death', and the above extracts provide descriptions of when these are present and when they are absent. It was clear that the presence of some kind of peace and acceptance helped not only the individual but also those who were present, whether family members or staff. Facilitating these aspects and as a result achieving a 'good death' for patients, family and staff was not necessarily an easy task, however. There were several dimensions to these features of a 'good death': for the organisation and professional staff, the family and the individual. These had a greater or lesser impact that depended on individual circumstances and the relationship between the patient, the family and the hospice.

Resolution

There was an expectation that the hospice could provide the opportunities to deal with 'unfinished business', to resolve difficulties and to have 'nothing left undone'.

> '*You know the other big thing I think about dying in here is that you have a huge opportunity to make your peace with everybody and you are encouraged in that... the majority of people who die don't die like this, say a heart attack or something, well then you don't have the opportunity. And it must be wonderful to know that you are dying and there is nothing left undone, in relationships and in personal terms, like if you fell out with your brother or your mother or whatever, you can make your peace now.*' (Elizabeth, administration, par. 152–4)

These expectations were sometimes unrealistic, however, as pre-existing family or personal difficulties could not always be resolved, and while palliative care professionals had very high standards, sometimes the expectations of the service were too high or unrealistic.

> '*I think we often set ourselves very high standards and I think the good death is a good death for everybody. We often have high expectations that we can provide support for families that have a huge amount of distress in the past. That the patient can have a good death with the resolution of possibly conflict or reconciliation with particular individuals and yet at the same time the family adjust to the impending death. But often at the same time we are dealing with the pre-existing conflicts and tensions that the social group, the family, have and often that is with the patient. So there is a period of heightened or more intense emotion in what is already a fairly fragile unit and then we try to do everything we can to make this right, or as right as it can be for all these people. And it's a pretty tall order.*' (Colm, social worker, par. 121)

This perception that the palliative care services can alleviate pain and psychological distress and provide support for the patient and the family may be problematic if these expectations are not fulfilled.

> '*People have expectations and is the hospice partly feeding these expectations in terms of, not in terms of saying this is a good death,*

> *but in terms of saying things, people shouldn't die in pain, and we can provide care that helps with psychological distress and support. But people may look back and say the hospice, all my relatives died in hospice and everyone was psychologically stressed and they sold themselves as being able to deal with it.'* (Margaret, doctor, par. 124)

For professional staff, not being able to achieve these aims and meet expectations caused personal difficulty, even though, realistically, they were aware of the potential problems in meeting the expectations. Deirdre talked about her emotional response to difficulties with some families while at the same time having to be realistic about what can be done.

> '*I suppose emotionally as well if the family find it difficult to let go, things have not been resolved, things like that can be hard because your heart goes out to them. And yet it can be hard maybe to resolve arguments that happened, you know, in the family maybe fifteen or twenty years ago that were never resolved, even when he was well.*' (Deirdre, nurse, par. 101)

Health care professionals may also have their own need for issues to be resolved, derived from a motivation to 'fix things', particularly before death.

> '*We have an agenda of our own. "He's not talking to his daughter, maybe he needs to make up with the daughter before he dies". I think what brings us into health care, I think all of us who go into health care have a need to help and to fix. We are "fixer-uppers" and we kind of like a happy ending. So it is all neat and tidy at the end. But we forget that these people come to this situation with their whole life experience and lives of interaction.*' (Emer, nurse, par. 87–9)

'Unfinished business'

Resolving 'unfinished business' seemed to be part of the preparation for a 'good death'. I had wondered whether this focus was one that originated with the professional staff rather than with patients, but Sheila, one of the doctors at St Theresa's, felt that, in her experience, the impetus to put some order on things generally came from patients. She likened it to preparation prior to any change, and talked about how, when changing jobs or taking a break from work, the impending change provided a focus and a deadline to tackle pieces of work that may have been present for quite a while.

Death and dying are, however, events of a different magnitude, and the kind of 'putting things in order' that is required is more complex and interwoven with the perceived needs of those who are living as well as those of the dying person. Some of the nursing staff and the chaplains talked about helping patients with these tasks in a somewhat formal way, such as letter-writing and creating memory banks for family members.

> '*They have been able to get unfinished business done, sometimes you might have written letters to people with them when they were kind of well. If you had a relationship with them that you could broach that subject and talk to them about, you know writing things down. And they would have done and in a sense it is good for them to do this and to know that they were leaving something behind. That if there were things you wanted to say, they were able to say them in writing. They wouldn't be writing, I would be writing it for them and they might sign the end of it, you know.*' (Pauline, chaplain, par. 41)

Putting things in some kind of order also happened informally and spontaneously, without intervention or facilitation from professionals.

> '*When she realised that she was not going to get better she actually just sat down and talked to us as regards how to be with one another. Like her house, all that would have to be organised and she didn't want us to fight over because she had seen so many families fighting over selling houses and things like that. We were able to say what we felt about her, and she said how good we were.*' (Monica, administration, par. 98)

Nevertheless, not all of the professional staff shared a view that resolving 'unfinished business' was a good thing to do.

> '*Some of the patients could deal with it okay if we would only let them, if they are happy to motor on and not discuss it, well, that's their privilege but I don't like this gut stuff, you know, digging in and trying to find out what is in there. Because you could open a can of worms with someone who is vulnerable and near death anyway and I am not into that much.*' (Angela, nurse, par. 65)

Some staff members felt that there was too much attention paid to trying to fix things, an attention the dying person did not always welcome.

> '*It's something I feel very strongly about because I'm a private person myself and I feel that a lot of time there can be too much prying going on into families and situations. There is always this thing of trying to fix situations and trying to solve situations. ... It just wouldn't be my approach. I'll try and build up a level of trust with somebody and then it's up to them to come back to me and say look, this is bothering me or I want to talk about this. You can over-hassle people, there have been a few comments recently from patients that like—if one more person asks me that question—you know.*' (Noirin, nurse, par. 157)

Acceptance

Acceptance of the inevitability of death appeared to be an important step in achieving a 'good death' for both the dying person and the family members. Reaching a point of acceptance, however, was dependent on being aware that death was going to happen, but there was a distinction between accepting death and being happy about it.

> '*The whole thing of accepting death phase, I am not sure exactly what acceptance means when you are talking about death and I think that sometimes drives people to unrealistic aims ... accepting death in recognising that it's going to happen, or accepting death as in welcoming it.*' (Sheila, doctor, par. 38)

Religious beliefs or a belief in an afterlife may not necessarily play a part in reaching acceptance as it may be more to do with acknowledging that this life is ending, whatever may lie ahead.

> '*I would feel he had a "good death"; a friend was asking him "Well, you know people when they are near death often have this sense of an afterlife and had he had any sense of this?" It was shortly before he died and he said "No he hadn't but he felt that this life had been good enough for him and that he was ready to face whatever was there". And I think it may be that you may have a strong belief that there is heaven and you are going to meet etc. but it may be that just you are ready for whatever.*' (Kevin, social worker, par. 76)

Reaching acceptance may be possible without any thought about or belief in what may come afterward.

> '*I have had a good life and this is the end of it, rather than I am looking forward to something good after it.*' (Sheila, doctor, par. 38)

Acceptance may also involve acknowledging that hopes and plans for the future are not realistic and recognising the value of the life that has been lived, although this may be particularly difficult in some instances.

> '*This patient had had alcohol addiction, had made his family angry for many years although he couldn't help it. He was saying "I have put that behind and now that I am free of that and wanting to live well and make it up to my family, because I have been such trouble. I am not going to get the rest of my life, it's being taken away just when I have got it back". He didn't know he was going to be ill when he went through the programmes, getting well. He had been cheated of having good quality time and giving back, but by the time he died he was saying "But I made a lot of people happy. My friends at the pub, we had great craic and the football, when I worked in England years ago, didn't we have a wonderful time?" And didn't we do this and didn't we do that, and I am*

> *wondering whether it is a survival thing in us, people start dropping the things that they had planned and can't do and at some stage there is a shift. A shift takes place and they say "Oh bugger all, I've had it", you know?'* (Joan, social worker, par. 63)

The cessation of treatment for illness and the handing over of the patient to palliative care services sometimes facilitated an acceptance that death was inevitable, but not all family members reached acceptance at the same time.

> *'She has changed. Now there are some things we can do about her changes, but she has changed and deteriorated. She had been back to the oncologist with her husband, last week. On the appointment before the oncologist had said he would give her oral chemotherapy. This visit there is no mention of oral chemotherapy. The oncologist said "The hospice will look after you". When he said it she had no problem, as she said herself, "Why should I go through that chemotherapy", she had dreadful side-effects. "It might give me three months but I might have three months extra of pain". And her little husband sat there and I said to him "You have questions too, would you need to go back and see the consultant?" And he said "No, no". And we came round then and we were talking about, you know, I can't remember how the conversation came around but then I said to him "You know she doesn't have a problem with where she is at the moment but you have anxieties around that". She was there and she said "Yes he does, yes he has, I have to go first, if I was left I couldn't cope, I couldn't cope, couldn't write a cheque, can't do the bank, I know nothing" and the poor man is there, you know, tortured. At the front door, he broke down and cried. And the only thing I could say to him was "I understand" because they are married thirty years, you don't wipe that out.'* (Sally, nurse, par. 57–9)

Acceptance also appeared to be reached by the dying person as they became more physically comfortable and peaceful, but not by family members, although death was very close.

> *'I would say for her family and for herself, she has been dying for a few days and before the point where you could really see she*

was changing and beginning to die—she had about four days where she was in a semiconscious state and yesterday she became unconscious. Before that, she really struggled with the whole separation from her family. She has really struggled with that, as have her family. This woman is in her fifties, the family would be in their late twenties, early thirties. They are both struggling with accepting that this is the actual end. But in the last twenty-four hours she is more comfortable and she is in a deep unconsciousness now. So hopefully in this time they can come to some sense of letting go a little bit. But it is really hard, I would say that this has been a real difficult death rather than a "good death".' (Christine, nurse, par. 22–6)

Acceptance was difficult when death occurred at what seemed an inappropriate stage in life. Many of the people I spoke with had difficulty accepting the death of a young person or a person with young children as in any way a 'good death'.

'*It would be hard to think of a "good death" in any context with a young person. If you were leaving behind young children ... how do you let go to die because you know you are leaving them ... that must be a terrible thing to come and have to give up yourself.*' (Jean, administration, par. 52)

When, however, death came at what was considered an appropriate stage of life—at the end of a life fully lived and when the time seems right—acceptance seemed easier.

'*I think older people sometimes; they just have more of an acceptance. ... We were looking after a woman in a nursing home and she was in her nineties, an amazing lady. She just decided she was going to die and I remember I was called down on the Friday, now she had become weaker but you would look at her and say, weeks, but definitely not soon. She called in the whole family and she told them she was going to die, she'd had enough you know, her husband was gone, her children were fine, they were well able to look after themselves, they had their own families and she was just tired, tired of living, tired of being here. She was ready to go and she died the following Tuesday. She just slipped away, no syringe driver, no symptoms, no nothing.*' (Lorraine, nurse, par. 91–3)

A continuum

Death may also be considered as part of a continuum, as moving from one set of relationships to another. Some dying people experienced the presence of deceased family members close to the time of death; for some patients this brought comfort and a sense that they were moving from one world to another, and they would not be alone. Margaret observed that, although some dying patients when they were close to death actually had a visual perception of someone deceased, it was more common for dying people to become aware, on some level, of people they had known who were already deceased.

> '*My experience would be as people get closer to death, not necessarily the dying moments, I hear them more experience people they know close at hand.*' (Margaret, doctor, par. 172)

Experiencing the presence of those already deceased brought acceptance and a sense of anticipation for some patients.

> '*My aunt of seventy-nine was diagnosed with cancer. And I remember I was doing the bereavement work* [educational course], *she was down in the hospital. So I had been doing the bereavement and all the care of the dying and I said, well, I am going to help her and get her to come to terms with her dying. ... she told me about her diagnosis and I remember saying to her "How do you feel?" She turned round to me and said "I can't wait". I said "What do you mean?" And she said "I am sitting here and I am having conversations with my twin" and all her sisters who had died before her. She was in that other place and communicating, this was real for her, with her friends, her sisters.... And I said to myself, "Well, nobody has to talk to you about acceptance". She couldn't, it wasn't that she couldn't wait but that she was ready and she was in that other halfway place where they had come and she was ready for her next adventure and I will never forget that.*' (Sally, nurse, par. 31)

Although not all dying people experienced people they knew close at hand, it was a common enough experience for professional staff to consider these experiences, however they may be understood, as one of the signs that death is relatively close.

> '*People seeing dead relatives, that is extremely common ... like, at this stage if somebody is seeing dead relatives like they are, I assume they are fairly close* [to death].' (Sheila, doctor, par. 137)

While it may be difficult to understand these experiences, they did seem to bring a sense of relief to both the dying person and the family members.

> '*There have been experiences here where people have had those kinds of sensations, where they have literally described who visited them; that they were relatives from previous generations. We have had an occasion here when somebody described somebody that they didn't know and it was a young woman; when her mother listened to the description she told her who it was. I suppose we hear them too often not to take them seriously so I would have an open mind around it, what that experience is. Some people might say it is drug-induced but some of the factors around, you know, some of the descriptions are quite clear. You know it can bring a great sense of relief to many people.*' (Colm, social worker, par. 149)

While the dying person may find these experiences a comfort, they were sometimes difficult for family members to understand and sometimes caused distress.

> '*I can think of some relatives who weren't so sure, in other words, when they talk about it like "My mother is now talking about seeing so and so", you know, who has been dead for years and they seem upset by that. They seem to think this is odd, it's weird, whereas the patient wouldn't report that, the patient would be very happy. The patient would report seeing them and would be unconcerned and unworried by it, some of them would actively say, would be pleased, comforted by it because they feel they are going to meet these people they have missed.*' (Margaret, doctor, par. 180)

Peace

A peaceful death seemed to be synonymous with a 'good death', but it was a particularly intangible aspect, as what appeared to bring a sense of peace to one person could also be what distressed another. Nevertheless, a sense of peace was something that seemed to come for most people at the end of the dying process.

> '*I only came across one man who fought with himself to the bitter end but ninety-nine per cent of people I have seen have had their struggles but they have died peacefully.*' (Christine, nurse, par. 92)

While resolution and acceptance seemed to be steps towards a peaceful death, there were also steps towards peace that involved a removal of anxiety, such as fears about the physical experience of death. Yet, while knowledge about the physical experience of death may have removed fear for some people, it was the cause of fear and anxiety in others.

> '*Some people are comforted by hearing that they are just going to get slowly weaker and weaker and going to sleep and then a deep sleep and then a coma, and pass away. Some will say "Oh it's like going to sleep, well that's fine". Others now have a difficulty sleeping at night because they are now fearful that they won't wake up.*' (Margaret, doctor, par. 41)

As already highlighted in the previous chapter, religious beliefs were sometimes problematic rather than helpful, and in the final days and hours this difficulty increased. Although a sense of peace was sometimes attained through religious beliefs and practices this was not always the case. For some people who had led lives with a strong religious conviction and practice, a lessening of the certainty of religious beliefs brought considerable distress.

> '*Often you would see people here who you would say have had a good death and they have great religious faith and peace within themselves. Now some people can be very religious but toward the end it is not a good death, there is a lot of fear, and anxiety and guilt and there is fifty medals pinned on to the nightdress and there is a huge anxiety. I have seen people who have been very involved*

> *in spirituality and prayer groups and all that sort of thing and come in here and had the most anxious time coming up to death.'* (Laura, nurse, par. 27)

On the other hand, some dying people turned to religious practice although this practice may not have been part of their lives.

> '*Even some people that never wished to have a priest, never wish to have anything and coming near the end they really want them but they get, you know, they get a sense of peace from them.*' (Lorraine, nurse, par. 75)

The individual 'good death'

A 'good death' was both an individual experience and, at the same time, an experience that belonged to other people. As an individual experience it was also unique.

> '*First of all we have to recognise that dying is a very individual thing. It's unique, no two people approach their death or in fact approach illness in the same way.*' (Emer, nurse, par. 32)

A 'good death' encompassed more than the physical experience of illness and death and involved a social relationship in which the individual's needs and desires were known.

> '*A good death would be if a patient got their wishes. If a patient wanted to die at home, I would be happy, if they wanted to die listening to music as somebody did recently, and they did, I would be happy. If they wanted to die with family around them, not with family around them, whatever their wishes are, that to me is a good death as opposed to sort of a medical thing. If we can do as much as they want, actually knowing, a good death to me is knowing what somebody would want.*' (Noirin, nurse, par. 78)

The dying person may wish to die without family members and sometimes this happened in ways that family members found difficult to accept.

> *'I have seen relatives sit for twenty-three hours, fifty-nine minutes and the one minute they have left the room, they go. I have said to people, if it is meant to be, if you are meant to be there, that's okay but you are not, you were not meant to be there neither. The person just has control and I don't want to say it will be how he lived but some people are very private and they will die on their own. And some people want everyone around them so I always say when you look back later on you will see that it was all meant to be that way.'* (Sally, nurse, par. 173)

Sometimes the dying person wished to exert control over the manner in which they died, and while this may have conflicted with acceptable levels of pain control or other aspects of care, some professional staff understood that by accepting the patient's wishes they were facilitating a 'good death', although it may have conflicted with their own views.

> *'If somebody does it the way they want to do it, you know, I mean, some people even want to sit in the chair and don't want to go to bed, they are allowed to do it the way they want to do it and that is what I consider a good death. You know, somebody might be very distressed by pain but they may be used to that and that might not be a major thing with them but they die the way they lived their lives and it is what they want to do and the way they want to do it.'* (Marie, nurse, par. 22)

Another aspect of facilitating patient autonomy and ultimately a 'good death' was apparent in accepting that the surroundings or the physical environment may not be providing comfort.

> *'Sometimes people will not want to be here, they will go home from here because they can come from what you might call chaotic surroundings but it would be more comfortable for them to be in those kind of surroundings.'* (Sheila, doctor, par. 40)

Not being closely involved with the patient and the family may also facilitate a 'good death'.

> *'People often die at home without any involvement from us. This is lovely to see as well, you know, they can die the way they live. I mean for a lot of them it just happens, and it is just helping the family to leave them to do it the way they want to do it.'* (Marie, nurse, par. 16)

Being able to die the way you wanted was a source of celebration for some family members.

> *'There was one family that, you know, said, he did it the way he wanted to and they were happy about it, and the doctor was saying that there was singing and laughing in the house the day he died, he did it the way he wanted to.'* (Marie, nurse, par. 188)

For some palliative care professionals, however, the exertion of control by the patient over the circumstances of death was uncomfortable, although the discomfort was recognised as one that was experienced by the observer rather than the dying person.

> *'Maybe for them it was a "good death", but for me looking on it wasn't. I remember a man came in and he never took his clothes off and he sat there dying on the chair. You wanted to take him and put him in the bed but no, he was doing it the way he wanted to. ... Sometimes our need to make it good for you or to make it the best it can be is because we can't deal with it, I can't deal with it, looking at you struggling in there to die, because it's not easy.'* (Pauline, chaplain, par. 23–5)

Knowing the dying person well enough prior to death was considered important in reaching an understanding of whether a death was good for a particular person.

> *'A "good death" is very much an individual thing and what I might consider as a bad death for somebody might in actual fact have been a very good death for the family. We can be subjective as well, in what we think of as "good death". I know a man who died yesterday; he looked as if he had a fantastic death, certainly from having seen him over the last six months and having known*

> *him. I would have said, if he was able to look back he would have said "Yes that was great, I slipped away so easily, I was walking the day before, I was out in the garden", he really didn't want to start losing his ability to do things for himself. On the other hand, his son missed his death but that may have been appropriate because he actually found it difficult when he came in and yet he was in the night before, had seen him and had seen a bit of a change in him.*' (Christine, nurse, par. 188–90)

Die as you live

A 'good death' was also considered to be one in which the attributes or values of the dying person were understood and reflected. Sometimes this was present in a positive way.

> '*You can often almost tell before people get to the dying stage, the little bit that we get to know about their lives and you see the way they relate to their family, and if there is a sense of peace and harmony and genuine caring and love then things tend to go okay.*' (Laura, nurse, par. 27)

People who were dying maintained their personal attributes and modes of behaviour, which did not necessarily change with the dying process.

> '*I feel people die as they live, you know, how can you expect somebody that kept everything to oneself all their lives at this really most important moment to change and become different.*' (Bernadette, chaplain, par. 184)

For some of the professional staff, the acceptance of the limitations of the palliative care model and an acknowledgment that not everything could be solved for each individual, and in a sense understanding the patients' perspective, facilitated a 'good death'.

> '*I think you die the way you have lived. If you have lived with turmoil all your life there is no way you can turn around and fix it. Sometimes you can, but you can't always expect to fix it in the*

> *end. I think it is acknowledging with the families that we can't fix it, that is the way he has done it and that is the way he wants to do it and that is fine, it could be a good death for them because that is the way they have lived.'* (Marie, nurse, par. 198)

The social 'good death'

Death is both an individual and a social experience that affects not only family members but also professional staff and the organisation.

Whose 'good death'?

Finding a balance between the individual experience and the experience of death for both family and staff was difficult as there was a potential conflict of needs and expectations from these different perspectives.

> *'I think I would like my death to be quick, which is a bit unfair on those I leave behind. Death is always good for you and it is back to what is a "good death"? Well it's a good death because that is what I want whereas you want me to linger on because then we can have these great chats, telling each other how we really feel about one another, but I am having a miserable time dying slowly.'* (Margaret, doctor, par. 95)

Palliative care professionals also had expectations of what a 'good death' was, especially in relation to the management of pain.

> *'This is where a conflict comes in then about what do patients want, what do families want and what do staff want? If somebody says "I don't want drugs because I want to be conscious", how do you fit with that? Palliative care staff can find it very difficult to accept that people can choose not to have pain relief.'* (Sheila, doctor, par. 52)

The view of whether or not a death was a 'good death' came from the perspective of the family members and professional staff rather than the person who died.

> *'You are not just trying to provide a "good death" for the person dying, ideally you are and the patient is our number one person. However, the only people reporting back to you are other people. I think this whole idea of a "good death" is a funny one when you look at it because who do we use to judge whether somebody had a good death, we do not use the patient we use the relatives.'* (Margaret, doctor, par. 89)

The emotional force of the death itself may have influenced the perception of family members.

> *'What I or other members of staff might have considered as a very comfortable death can be experienced by family members as horrific, as a very painful struggle for the person and clearly all the other evidence would point to a very peaceful experience of death for the patient. But the perception of the surviving friend or relative is that it was a terrible, desperate experience and what can often happen is that there is a projection of the power and desperation of the actual reality of the loss and the devastation of that into the arena of the actual dying experience.'* (Colm, social worker, par. 75)

Managing a 'good death'

The needs of the patient and the needs of the family certainly influenced each other and at times conflicted. This interplay between the dying person and family members and the needs of staff required careful management by the professional staff. The management of the physical and social space within the in-patient unit at St Theresa's was already discussed in Chapter 6. The management of family members and the dying patient became more complex during the final days and hours, and sometimes this was exacerbated by the frequent presence of large families in an environment where there were other dying people and their families present.

> *'In some families, for a start there is a huge number and particularly at night, they are asked to wait outside, not wait outside, but two at a time because people might want to sleep or whatever. But a lot of people might want to actually be there and*

> *some people might have eleven in the family. They might sit outside and then they would go in and out. We try to, when someone is actually dying, because of the heat of the room, to ask people to do it in relays you know.'* (Angela, nurse, par. 158)

Palliative care professionals have the experience and knowledge of the physical aspect of dying which may have appeared painful and uncomfortable to the family members; sharing this knowledge with family members sometimes reduced distress.

> *'If a patient has been very chesty, now they may be semi-unconscious or practically unconscious but it sounds to the family as if the patient is drowning and that they're aware of it. So we would always say to the families, you know that while it's difficult for you sitting here listening to this, you know, but he is not distressed by that, he wouldn't be aware and that he is not drowning and that he is peaceful.'* (Deirdre, nurse, par. 101)

Managing the emotional impact of the physical experience of death was often difficult for staff as they were also aware that the dying person was sometimes aware of the tension.

> *'What I might perceive as a good death the patient's family might think is absolutely horrific. As a nurse, what I hope would be that a patient is relaxed, symptoms well managed and peaceful, a peaceful death. But in the course of that they might get, a lot of patients get chesty towards the end and that could be very distressing to the family and they cannot cope. They say "Listen to him, it is horrific, he is choking". They cause us a huge amount of anxiety, and you are trying to keep it calm around the bed and often this anxiety is very high. The patient can feel it and it does get tense, it does unsettle them and it is how to manage that as best you can. It might be just a couple of times but with a few different staff members, you could find a way of saying "This is quite normal, they are not distressed".'* (Geraldine, nurse, par. 86)

The dying person may also have been aware of difficult family dynamics, which sometimes increased anxiety and restlessness.

> *'If there is an argument going on within the family unit itself that one sister mightn't be talking to the other or things like that can be very awkward. You would have families that could be fighting with each other over the bed. You would have to bring them aside and say while your father is asleep or unconscious he may be aware, he may be drifting in and out of different levels of consciousness, you know you can't be speaking over the bed like that, but in a sensitive way.'* (Deirdre, nurse, par. 101)

Getting the balance right between family needs and patient needs was a difficult task for the staff.

> *'A case that we have at the moment it is a very difficult situation. They are in on top of their mother continuously, they will come out and say she is restless, she is very anxious. Yet when we are with her, she is actually very relaxed because the family have stood back, so when they go back in again she becomes restless again. You can't tell the family that they can't stay and they can't visit, it is very difficult.'* (Geraldine, nurse, par. 90)

Harmonious death

A peaceful death or a 'good death' may also be regarded as a death that is in harmony with the life that has been lived, with the personal qualities of the dying person, and with the process and events that surrounded the death and with a natural cycle of life and death.

Dying the way one wanted to die may have its own resonance with the dying person and family, and this may have brought a sense of peace.

> *'We had a young girl come in, she was only in her early twenties, but she had been diagnosed and they had offered her chemo, they'd offered her loads of treatments and she said no, she went off travelling around the world and then died very peacefully afterwards and very happily and the family very happy about it.'* (Noirin, nurse, par. 143)

A harmonious flow with the process of dying and the surrounding events seemed to bring a sense of a peaceful death.

> '*Before I came into palliative care, somebody that I knew died and I always thought she died well. Her family and I were at the bedside and her son-in-law was there and her daughter as well, and her sister. She waited for her son to come from America and he did. I remember thinking then on that day, gosh, I will never be afraid of death again in my life, she had a peaceful death, she just didn't struggle and her family all got there, all the way from America.*' (Angela, nurse, par. 56)

A death may also be in harmony with the dying process where the dying person and the family have accepted death, and when death comes it is a peaceful end to the process.

> '*I looked after this elderly man, he had a big family and his wife was alive, very supportive and very close. From the day he came in he was religious, and from the day he came in he was saying he knew he was here to die and he was happy and he had made his peace and he had lived his life to the full and everything was positive. It went like that all the way through, and the evening he died he was still conscious up until the moment he died and I remember I went in to him about fifteen minutes before he died, and I asked him if he was okay and he opened his eyes a little bit and said "I am very happy". It was wonderful for the family who were all around him. That obviously has to do with his personality but also there is the whole thing about how he lived his life as well.*' (Laura, nurse, par. 84)

A sense of death as part of a continuum and not as an ending may bring a sense of harmony, for staff and family members.

> '*I have experienced on night duty, it always stayed with me, it's nearly three years now. Looking after an elderly gentleman at night, his three daughters were around the bed, his wife had gone home and we had promised her that if we felt we saw a change, we would have her called back. This gentleman, he let the most beautiful smile out of him about two minutes before he died. He*

> *literally opened his eyes, now he was in a deep unconscious, he opened his eyes, smiled; the smile lasted about twenty seconds. That smile has always remained with me, it was almost that he had seen something; you didn't want to go away from the bedside.... In that case there was a sense that this man had gone beyond and had given us a slight glimpse because that is three years ago and it's still as plain as anything and the whole situation around it, even when his wife came in. There was a sense of, a real sense of calmness and peace.*' (Christine, nurse, par. 110)

Religious beliefs about an afterlife may shape how this continuum is understood and received.

> '*He very much had a sense of the spiritual although he was in no way an overtly pious kind of a man and he had had a difficult time, he had had a lot of pain to control and he had had a lot of suffering. His family were there and his wife described herself as being to one side of him and her daughter at the other. Then the priest came and when it became clear that he was actually dying the priest moved aside to let his daughter stand by her father's bedside and he moved down to the end of the bed and they were praying. His wife said she had this perception of him being received in a heavenly situation and of the prayers being continued in a heavenly setting.*' (Carol, doctor, par. 142)

Finally, dying may also be seen as death that is in harmony with the natural cycle of life and death and of nature.

> '*There was a man that died and there were doors out to the garden and I pushed his bed out because he wanted to feel the sun on his face and the family were just sitting around the bed and the grandchildren came into the garden beside him, just sitting there and he died. It was just so, it was so spiritual, or just so at one with nature— in the sun, the cycle of day and night and of life and death.*' (Catherine, nurse, par. 126)

Summary

This chapter has considered how a 'good death' was understood and shows that a 'good death' is dualistic, having both individual and social dimensions. The individual dimension was always intensely personal, the understanding of which was enhanced by a relationship with the dying person. The social dimension of a 'good death' incorporated the needs of family and also of staff and the organisation. A 'good death' was a death that was in harmony with these elements.

SECTION 3
CREATING SOCIAL MAPS:
UNDERSTANDING THE TOPOGRAPHY

INTRODUCTION

Mapping has been a central theme in this research and, following Elias's identification of blank areas in the social map of death and dying, this final section utilises cartography to create a social map of death and dying in an Irish hospice setting. This section presents the 'key' or legend to the preceding section. Section 2 has largely described the experience of palliative care in Ireland in the specific location of St Theresa's Hospice and has moved through a series of 'maps' or sketches toward a more detailed view of a 'good death'. This final section draws these sketches together and provides, through consideration of the social and political contexts and the theoretical perspectives of Elias and Foucault, a way of understanding the social landscape of the care for the dying in Ireland.

Chapters 4–6 in section 2 have described the research setting and how the key aspects of palliative care—open awareness, communication, total pain and multi-disciplinary working—discussed in Section 1 are worked out in the context of a palliative care service in Ireland. It is clear that this service is shaped and influenced by the historical context of Catholicism in Ireland, in the lives of the citizens and in the workings of the health care structures and organisations. Chapters 7 and 8 have presented a detailed view of spiritual care and a 'good death'.

It is evident that the spiritual care dimension of palliative care was considered as larger than, but encompassing, religious beliefs and practice. Spirituality appeared, from the views of participants, to be an essential core of the person; part of that core may or may not include religion. Spiritual care was considered as a role of accompaniment facilitated by a personal relationship between staff and the patient.

Religious practice and belief remain important for many people, and some people return to religious practice at the end of life. Nevertheless, it is also clear that religious practice and belief can be problematic. Part of the problem was the past experience of the Catholic Church in the lives of the patients, although some elements of the belief system, a belief in a judgemental God, for instance, inducing feelings of fear and guilt, also caused problems.

A 'good death' was considered to have two separate but interwoven aspects—individual and social. It was clear that while the individual aspects of a 'good death' were always unique, the social aspects, which include the dying person, the family and the staff, can be understood more generally. The aspects of a 'good death' that are well documented in the literature and which also formed part of this research such as resolution, acceptance and peace have a direct impact on the perception of a social 'good death' and all form aspects of the 'manner of parting', as discussed in Chapter 1.

The theme of relationship is a central one to emerge from this research. The person-centred approach of palliative care has aided the formation of relationships: however, it also raised questions about their nature and about the cultural context in which they are located. Relationships between the professional staff and the patient and the family all formed elements of the social aspect of a 'good death' and were shaped by the 'manners' of social engagement and the location of care—at home, in the day care centre and in the in-patient unit.

A relationship also exists between the palliative care services, the health care service in Ireland, the Catholic Church and the larger cultural context. Culture cannot be separated out as a distinct strand, although it is visible in some of the cultural differences that were discussed in Section 1 and also highlighted by some of the participants in the research. Cultural practices and ways of behaving are deeply embedded in the social fabric, however, which in turn is located in a historical context. The influence of the Catholic Church in health care and other social institutions was highlighted in Chapter 2. Although the involvement of the Catholic Church has greatly diminished, it has left a legacy that has shaped the Ireland of today.

This section will examine the 'maps' or chapters from Section 2 that were laid out for view. Chapter 9 will consider the underlying topography—that is, the relationship between palliative care services, the health care service and the role played by groups within the Catholic Church and the medical professions in shaping these services. It will discuss the historical legacy that has shaped the current service, which in turn provides a foundation for the future. It will examine whether, as Keegan and van Doorslaer (2001) have argued, the Ireland of today is characterised by a changing landscape in which more than one reference or guide is used and, if so, what these references are and their current visibility. It will also consider the understandings of a 'good death' and definitions of spiritual care.

Chapter 10 will consider the relationships that occur within the topography discussed in Chapter 9 and will develop an understanding of these in relation to Elias's figurational approach and Foucault's observations of the dynamics of power. It will identify the presence of fine lines between lay and professional perspectives, fine lines that need to be negotiated with skill and balance. Of significance here is the role of the researcher and the fine lines that must be negotiated in a research setting. In this context the nature of ethical decision-making in qualitative research is revisited, together with a discussion of the reflexive process.

CHAPTER 9
A complex relationship

Introduction

Keegan and van Doorslaer (2001) have considered a changing landscape in which more than one explanation or guide is used as a reference for behaviour as characteristic of contemporary Ireland. Taylor (1989) has stated that death is a potent time for important issues in a culture to be made visible, suggesting that the dynamics involved in this changing landscape will be more visible in practices and beliefs around death and dying.

The involvement of religious orders in health care and other social institutions is now much reduced; however, a Catholic religious order was highly influential in shaping the underlying organisational values at St Theresa's. The apparent 'naturalness' of religion in Ireland, an important aspect of the research, is due in part to the role of the Church in social institutions, and religion and religious discourse may be the main cultural language, although no longer the only one.

The practice of palliative care shapes a 'good death' and the type of spiritual care that forms part of the model of care; these aspects, however, cannot be separated from their cultural context, and while this is a new model of care, the context in which it operates is embedded in a pre-existing health care system and a set of cultural practices and beliefs.

The legacy of the past

In a discussion of the changing role of the NHS and palliative care in the UK, Small states that the NHS and palliative care exist within a complex relationship of what has been done in the past, what can be done in the present and what might be achieved in the future (2003, 20). While this is certainly true in the UK, a similar complex relationship exists in Ireland between the health care system, palliative care services and the role and position of the Catholic Church.

The organisational values at St Theresa's were in tune with the values of palliative care developed initially by Cicely Saunders within a Christian tradition of care. Palliative care in the UK has become part of the NHS and operates within that health care system, as discussed in Chapter 1. This incorporation, and the development of the medical specialism of palliative medicine, may have led to a diversification of the initial reformist agenda (James and Field 1992). Developmental challenges for palliative care continue within mainstream health care; the extension of services to non-cancer patient groups is one example. In the UK these developments take place within an equitable health service, although admittedly an overstretched and under-funded service.

In Ireland palliative care also faces challenges, but the context for these changes is within a fundamentally flawed health service that is also under-staffed and under-funded. Within the Irish health care system the type of palliative care service operated by the religious order at St Theresa's was a welcome and positive change from general health care, a health care system that has been fraught with ad hoc development and interference from powerful groups within medicine and the Catholic Church. The equity of service provided by St Theresa's that many of the participants in this research remarked upon and appreciated needs to be understood within the context of health care in Ireland.

The Irish health care system

The Irish health care system underpins the development and delivery of palliative care services in Ireland. It is a two-tiered system, incorporating both public and private health care, in a manner that has been described by the Organisation for Economic Co-operation and Development as 'unique' (OECD 1997, 116). Wren in an exhaustive analysis of the current health care system in Ireland suggests that this is a diplomatic description of a health service that could more accurately be described as 'bizarre' (2003, 16).

Public health care in Ireland is funded from general taxes, although it is not available to everyone in the same way. The poorest 30% of the population—and, since 2001, people over 70 years of age—are entitled to free medical treatment (under a General Medical Services scheme) with general practitioners and free medication. (This entitlement for people over 70 was decreased in the 2008 budget.) The remainder of the population pay for visits to family doctors and a large proportion of their medication. Private health insurance, which approximately 50% of the population subscribe to, funds a small part of the costs for GP services (*ibid.*, 16). Families on low income who do not qualify for a medical card and who cannot afford private health insurance may be unable to afford visits to general practitioners and medication.

The state funds the public hospitals, which can be state-run or under the control of voluntary groups, such as Catholic religious orders, similar to the way in which St Theresa's Hospice was funded. People who hold medical cards are entitled to free hospital treatment and the remainder of the population pay limited charges. Emergency cases are dealt with on a first-come basis, but access to all other hospital services is through a slow public waiting list that can entail waiting years for some treatments.

Although waiting lists are present in the NHS in the UK, in September 2002 in the UK three patients in every 10,000 had waited over a year, while in Ireland the figure is 21 adult patients per 10,000 of the population. For those who can afford private health insurance it is possible to receive treatment within days or weeks, in publicly funded hospitals. This position is again in contrast with the NHS, where, although pay beds for private patients exist, they constitute only 1% of total NHS admissions. In the UK approximately 11% of the population have some form of private health insurance; in Ireland in 2001 that figure was 46% (*ibid.*, 331).

An unusual aspect of the Irish health care system is, according to Wren (2003), the manner in which private and public care is combined. Public hospital consultants receive extra payment for each private patient treated. In addition to receiving state salaries, consultants may also work in private hospitals. This system provides an economic incentive for consultants to treat private patients, which in turn contributes to public waiting lists (*ibid.*, 17). A recent report (*Commission on Financial Management and Control Systems in the Health Service*: Government of

Ireland 2003) has stated that the 'existing arrangements for mixing public and private treatments are inherently unsatisfactory from a management and control perspective. They result in a conflict of interests for Consultants between meeting clinical obligations to public patients on the one hand, and, on the other, the prioritisation, treatment and the use of publicly provided infrastructure and resources in public hospitals for private patients' (*ibid.*, 71).

In addition to an inequitable health care system, the public hospitals have been consistently under-funded and under-resourced; for instance, in spite of a rise in population over a twenty-year period, the number of acute hospital beds has fallen from 17,665 in 1981 to 11,985 in 2001 (Acute Hospital Bed Capacity Review, cited in Wren 2003). Health care systems in other countries, such as the NHS in the UK, also suffer from under-funding and under-resourcing, but the system is at least equitable. Wren has described the Irish system as a hybrid, combining elements of the UK and US health care systems in a 'unique mixture' (*op. cit.*, 18). The development of the health service and the influence of powerful lobbies were discussed in Chapter 2. Despite subsequent developments there have been no fundamental changes that have addressed the issue of equity.

The establishment of the health boards

The 1970 Health Act provided changes to the health care system, although these changes were largely administrative rather than addressing issues of equitable access to services. The only improvement in services was a drugs refund scheme whereby expenditure on medications over a certain threshold would be reimbursed by the health boards, irrespective of income (Wren 2003, 48). However, further concessions to the Catholic bishops and the medical consultants were made prior to the passing of the Act. The Minister permitted the voluntary hospitals to retain control of consultancy appointments, and hospitals run by the Catholic Church, which were the majority, were reassured that they could insist on Catholic ethics in medical practice, whatever the religious affiliation of patients or staff members (Barrington 1987, 272).

The Health Strategy 2001

In 2001 the Department of Health and Children published a comprehensive Health Strategy document—*Quality and fairness: a health system for you*—which has four stated goals: better health for everyone, fair access, responsive and appropriate care delivery and high performance. Allied to these goals are specific objectives that emphasise health promotion, equitable access for all categories of patients, a patient-focused approach, and a standardised quality system to support patient care (Department of Health and Children 2001, 58).

While the Health Strategy is laudable in its stated goals, it has been criticised by the United Nations Committee on Economic, Social and Cultural Rights as lacking a human rights framework. The panel of international health experts invited to advise the Department of Health and Children during the drafting of the strategy also argued for the 'establishment of health as a fundamental human right' and as a key starting-point for the strategy, from which 'full access to quality health services would follow' (Wren 2003). In spite of these arguments the Health Strategy contained no proposal to change the 30-year-old legislation.

A balancing view

An account of the historical development of the Irish health service, discussed in Chapter 2, clearly shows considerable influence from groups within both the Church and medicine; however, the Irish health service has also benefited enormously from innovations and investment by many Catholic religious orders since the nineteenth century. While the Catholic Church took on many of the functions of the state, as Inglis (1998) has demonstrated, and has shaped these services in a direction it desired, some religious orders, such as the Sisters of Charity, have been proactive and visionary in the services they have established—their work in establishing the initial palliative care services in Ireland was discussed in Chapter 2. The Daughters of Charity and other orders of religious nuns and brothers have been similarly proactive and innovative in establishing services for vulnerable groups, such as services for people with learning disability. Once established, these services have attracted state funding, but it has been the religious orders and not the state that have identified a need for services and that have made the initial investments in the infrastructure, the finances and the personnel.

Equity of service

Against the backdrop of what I have argued is a flawed and inequitable health care system it is not surprising that many of the participants appreciated the type of care that was available at St Theresa's. Sr Bridget and the religious order established equal access from the onset of the service, and current staff and management continued this commitment although the hospice would certainly have gained financially from private health insurance contributions, as other hospices have found. In the context of the level of influence brought to bear by politicians, the Church and other interest groups over the years, it is not surprising that the comment made by one doctor that political contacts for a bed in the hospice 'cuts no ice' received a welcome from staff.

While equitable access to the palliative care services at St Theresa's is deserving of praise, palliative care itself is not equitable as this is a service that has evolved and developed within cancer care, as discussed in Chapter 1, and is currently provided primarily for cancer patients, although small numbers of other restricted patient groups are facilitated. The ethics of this inequity have been debated in the palliative care literature (Addington-Hall and Higginson 2001), and this was discussed briefly in Chapter 1. In Ireland, some progress has been made toward the inclusion of other patient groups, such as people suffering from motor neurone disease, and this figure is approximately 2% of those cared for by the palliative care services (Igoe *et al.* 1997).

There are other patient groups who could benefit from the level of services that are available to cancer patients. People with dementia are considered one of a number of appropriate patient groups for palliative care (Addington-Hall and Higginson 2001). People suffering from dementia, as one example, represent a large and vulnerable patient group, and in Ireland the provision of care for people with dementia is poor. It is estimated that there are approximately 33,000 people with dementia, and just over 22,000 of these live in the community (Lawlor *et al.* 1994). In spite of this considerable number, the level of support for maintaining people with dementia in the community is almost non-existent. Most people with dementia are cared for at home, and very frequently by elderly spouses. Research has shown that family members caring for people with dementia bear considerable risks of mental and physical illness, social isolation and financial difficulties to a much greater extent than people not caring for dementia patients (Albinsson and Strang 2003). When people with dementia do need intensive nursing and residential placement, there are limited places within publicly funded care settings available in Ireland. A varying standard of unregulated private nursing home places are available at considerable cost, none of which provide the type of high-quality care and physical environment that were available at St Theresa's.

A culture of Catholicism

The historical involvement of the Catholic Church in social institutions in Ireland, discussed in Chapter 2, has led to the presence and influence of the Church in all aspects of social life. The influence of the Church has lessened in recent years and there is now a separation of Church and State. Other factors, such as the fall in vocations, already outlined, have resulted in the Catholic Church being unable to maintain its overriding presence. Inglis has argued that the control exercised by the clergy, even in their absence, resulted in the supervisory eye of the Church being internalised in the hearts and minds of Irish Catholics (1998, 211). This level of control and supervision has also lessened, as the presence of religious and clergy especially in education has become considerably diminished; nevertheless, it could be considered that this internalisation has led to the creation of a culture of Catholicism, the extent of which is not always immediately apparent.

Cultural features can be so hidden and taken for granted that they are difficult to identify. Inglis (1998) has argued that Ireland differs from other European and Catholic countries because in Ireland the Catholic Church fulfilled a role as the civilising influence in the formation of the state, a situation that did not occur elsewhere in Europe. In establishing social institutions such as schools and hospitals the Catholic Church became a major force in Irish society and a major influence and presence for citizens at all stages of life.

A very large percentage of Irish people are Roman Catholics, although the 2002 recent census figures show a decline in the percentage of Roman Catholics in Ireland. The actual number of Roman Catholics has risen during a ten-year period (1991–2002) by 7.3%; there has also been an increase in the population, however, and as the percentage increase was lower than the rise in the population as a whole over that period (11.1%), the number of Roman Catholics in the population fell from 91.6% in 1991 to 88.4% in 2002 (Central Statistics Office 2007). This census has also recorded sizeable increases in the numbers of Church of Ireland (Anglican), Presbyterian and Methodist members. This reverses a long-term decline, but the Central Statistics Office (2007) states that immigration is the principal reason for this increase, with a total of 27,000 immigrants stating that they belonged to one of these religions. The number of Muslims has also risen dramatically in this ten-year period, showing a 15.3% increase. This is also attributed to immigration (*ibid.*, 29). These changes in the religious affiliation of the population will have interesting and considerable implications for health care services in the future.

The naturalness of religion

In this study it was clear that St Theresa's Hospice was a Catholic place and organisation. One of the doctors in the study remarked that she was not now a Catholic but had been raised as one, and as such felt she was too close to see how Catholic St Theresa's might be. This comment mirrored my own experience, as prior to undertaking the research I had made a few visits to a hospice which had been established by another religious order. Since conducting the research my awareness of the apparent invisibility of a Catholic presence has been heightened, as on revisiting this hospice recently I was shocked by the number and prominence of religious images on show at almost every turn in the building (albeit an older part of the building, not the newer in-patient unit), but more shocked that I had not even noticed these previously.

One respondent in this study considered that religion was very 'natural' in Ireland. This sense of religion as being 'natural' may be due in part to the total coverage of social institutions by the Catholic Church so that at every stage of the life course, such as births, marriages and deaths, the Church has both a civil and religious function. For instance, not having children baptised into a Christian faith, Catholic or Protestant, can cause considerable difficulty, as almost all primary education for children is in the hands of either Catholic or Protestant schools. While non-allegiance to a Christian faith will not exclude children from these schools, their inclusion is not unproblematic in terms of being able to participate in the activities of the school. Religious education is part of the curriculum, and preparation for the first reception of the sacrament of Holy Communion in the Catholic Church, which takes place at around the age of seven, is an important social as well as religious event.

Davie (2000) has argued that a decline in institutional religion does not imply a decline in or disappearance of beliefs or spiritual practices, and identified what seems to be occurring as people 'believing but not belonging'. In Ireland this situation may be reversed: for instance, having children baptised as Catholic may have less to do with beliefs and allegiance and much more to do with a lack of choice and a decision to smooth the path of social interaction and integration, leading more to a case of 'belonging but not necessarily believing'.

A lack of choice was one issue highlighted by a doctor in this research who tried to put herself in the shoes of a patient coming into the hospice—'The only thing on a patient's mind might be that hospice care in the area is run by a religious order and they can talk all they like about spiritual but that's Catholic'; with limited palliative care services available, the majority of which are in the hands of Catholic religious orders, there is a real lack of choice. Respondents in this study also remarked that some patients who came into the in-patient unit refused initially to have anything to do with the chaplains but by the end were planning their funeral

Mass. While respondents seemed to feel that this was a return to religious practice and as such demonstrated that religious practice was important to people, it may have had more to do with social integration within the hospice in addition to smoothing the path for family members, especially as funerals are important social events in Ireland.

A lack of choice regarding chaplaincy services in health care settings in the UK has been discussed in Chapter 1 (Orchard 2001; Wright 2001), suggesting that lack of choice is not exclusive to Ireland. This lack of choice, however, relates to one aspect of the health care service. The role of chaplains and religious in health care settings and organisations in the UK may be considerably less than is the case, currently and historically, in Ireland; in addition, this lack of choice relates to one aspect of the service and not the entire service.

A Catholic discourse

An article in the *Sunday Times* highlighted the issues surrounding physician-assisted suicide and euthanasia (Brewis 2003). Drawing on high-profile cases such as that of motor-neurone sufferer Diane Pretty, who took her case to the European Court of Human Rights in 2002, Brewis documents a growing support for a change in the law. While this issue is publicly debated in the UK and the seminal journal for palliative care, *Palliative Medicine*, devoted a special issue to this debate in 2003, discussed below, very little debate has taken place in Ireland on this issue.

The European Association of Palliative Care (EAPC) Ethics Task Force have been addressing this issue since 2001 and present definitions of euthanasia and physician-assisted suicide (Materstvedt *et al.* 2003). They state that withholding futile treatment, withdrawing futile treatment and providing 'terminal sedation', i.e. the use of sedative medication to relieve intolerable suffering in the last days of life, should not be considered as euthanasia (2003, 98).

The Task Force acknowledge that several approaches to this issue are emerging in Europe and argue that ongoing debate should be encouraged. Nevertheless, they also highlight potential problems should euthanasia be legalised:

these include pressure being brought to bear on or perceived by vulnerable persons and the underdevelopment or devaluation of palliative care. The Task Force advocate that the EAPC should respect individual choices for euthanasia but should refocus attention on the responsibility of all societies to provide care for their elderly, dying and vulnerable citizens.

A similar view was expressed by Cicely Saunders in an editorial in this special issue of *Palliative Medicine*. Saunders argues that without statutory or voluntary palliative care services being offered, 'more and more people will find their lives not worth living and it will be society's indifference rather than any lack of potential that their lives still have that will lead them to ask for a "right to die"' (2003, 103).

This issue of *Palliative Medicine* drew contributions from palliative care professionals in 33 countries around the world. There was no contribution from palliative care professionals in Ireland. In 2001 a statement from the Irish Association of Palliative Care (O'Regan 2001) called for euthanasia to remain illegal and addressed the issue of caring for sick and vulnerable people, a view that reflects that of European palliative care. Some opinion pieces have appeared sporadically (O'Brien 2001; Myers 2003; Myers 2004) in addition to newspaper coverage that appeared at the time of an assisted suicide in Dublin in 2002 (Rae and Smyth 2002; Reilly 2002; Humphreys 2002). The Irish Episcopal Conference (Conference of Irish Roman Catholic Bishops) published a leaflet entitled *Living with dying*: a letter from the Irish bishops to mark the Day for Life, October 2002. This document explores the moral position of euthanasia and the use of drugs that may improve the quality of life but lead a person to die sooner owing to side-effects such as depression of breathing; it examines the use of these drugs under the moral principle of double effect. It states that their use is legitimate from a moral point of view provided that 'There is no intention to end the life of the person who is dying and the reduction in the patient's length of life is not out of proportion to the pain-relief that he or she experiences'.

The bishops' letter also emphasises that 'only God has the right to decide when a life should end' and that 'the sacraments of the Eucharist, of reconciliation and of anointing the sick have an important part to play as these sacraments are a way of bringing inner healing and strength to the person who is sick'. Palliative care, according to the bishops, 'facilitates good pastoral and sacramental care because it frees patients from excessive anxiety and pain'.

This document was distributed to all Catholic churches in October 2002 and is still available in many churches. None of the chaplains at St Theresa's professed any knowledge of its preparation and publication and seemed puzzled and not a little annoyed about the apparent lack of consultation with chaplains working in palliative care, although it would appear that advice from some palliative care professionals was sought. The production of this leaflet by the Catholic bishops indicates that the hierarchy of the Catholic Church consider their input and influence to be still considerable.

A cultural language

Communication is a key aspect of palliative care, as discussed in earlier chapters. Many of the professional staff, and nursing staff in particular, often spoke about 'inching forward' and 'listening for clues'. This tentative and often unspoken aspect of communication has already been discussed in relation to spiritual care and symbolic language (Stanworth 1997; Czechmeister 1994; Roy 1999).

It was clear that visible signs of a religious presence seemed important for some people—one of the doctors in the study remarked that for the age group that formed much of the patient group in the hospice, the presence of nuns and priests and the saying of prayers were important. Others in the study also talked about the comfort, strength and consolation that were derived from prayers and the sacraments, although this was not true of everyone, as already described.

One of the nurses in the study spoke of her experience of nursing in the UK, where prayers would have been said before or just after death. She felt, however, that in Ireland religion was a much more integrated part of people's 'journeys'. The metaphor of journeying is, of course, not uncommon in relation to death and dying, but it was frequently used and always in the sense of a journey toward God. A religious perspective formed part of everyday language. When talking about people who were about to die or who had just died, in day-to-day conversation people often said 'they are on their way to God' or 'they have gone to God'. Nurses spoke about saying 'gentle prayers to see him on his way'.

What was interesting from this study was the way in which prayers facilitated the communication component of palliative care. Prayers seemed to be a common way for nursing staff to manage communication with family members and served as an indicator that death was close without this being made explicit. At other times saying prayers provided the nursing staff with a chance for unobtrusive observation and opportunities to open up communication with family—as one nurse remarked, 'an opportunity to see how they were feeling'. Some prayers, such as the Rosary, were often said just after the death. This type of repetitive prayer has a meditative quality that can be soothing and can calm down heightened emotions. Prayers at the time of death were also perceived by one family member, as relayed to me by a member of staff, as 'being continued in a heavenly setting', prayers in this sense providing not only a sense of reassurance and comfort but a mechanism for continuing dialogue with the deceased.

Pilgrimage also offered a mechanism for establishing levels of awareness about the closeness of death—one home care nurse in the study spoke about her surprise at finding a daughter planning to take her father to Lourdes in September when it was clear to the nurse that he would probably not be alive in September. Pilgrimages to Lourdes were important to many people and, as staff remarked, brought peace and acceptance, not necessarily to the dying person but to family members.

An interesting aspect was the degree to which it was nursing staff and not the chaplains who talked about prayers, giving weight to Inglis's argument that Catholicism has been internalised in the hearts and minds of Irish Catholics. Bernadette, one of the chaplains, specifically said that she did not 'go in to pour prayers down but to be with the person'. Pauline, another chaplain, acknowledged that she had the expertise to talk about people's spiritual lives and prayers but also felt that all the staff could and did do this. The apparent naturalness of religion in Ireland is due to the fact that all the social institutions in Ireland, from the cradle to the grave, are shaped by religious institutions.

A changing landscape

Ireland has been characterised as a changing landscape (Keegan and van Doorslaer 2001) in which more than one explanation or guide is used as a reference for behaviour in relation to attitudes and beliefs around death and dying. Small (2003) argues that the way forward must take account of the past and the present for future developments in palliative care.

Hornsby-Smith and Whelan (1994) have argued that a new type of Catholic is emerging who displays an informed appreciation of the value of the supernatural and sacramental life of the Church, as well as an increasing tendency to think in terms of a spirit or life force rather than a personal God. Inglis (1998) has developed this further, arguing that Irish Catholics no longer see the Catholic Church as a moral authority and that there is a move toward Protestantism and the emergence of 'Protestant Catholics', as already outlined in Chapter 2.

This shift reflects earlier changes elsewhere. Rumbold (2002) has argued that the recent interest in spirituality runs counter to the expectations of the 1960s and 1970s social theorists who predicted an increase in secularisation in western societies. Secularisation theory was developed from studies of the decline of institutional religion, especially in European societies. Studies from North America and developing nations in Asia, Africa and South America have shown, however, that religion does not inevitably decline as a society develops technologically (2002, 13). Lyon (2000) has argued that what may have been interpreted as secularisation is actually a deregulation of religion, whereby beliefs and practices associated with religious institutions are no longer under their control but may be adapted by individuals. Berger (1997, 974) has stated that what he and other sociologists wrote in the 1960s about secularisation was a mistake and that 'most of the world today is certainly not secular...it's very religious'.

Rumbold (2002) has stated that from the seventeenth century, with the fragmentation of religious authority during the Renaissance and Reformation, religion became differentiated from culture. As religious authority declined, the authority of science increased. The dominance of science has been mediated through social institutions allied to science, and health care, according to Rumbold, is one example of this (*op. cit.*, 9). This may have been the case in Europe and elsewhere but it clearly was not the case in Ireland. The previous discussions have shown the degree to which Catholicism is embedded in Irish cultural practice. In addition, the Reformation and the development of Protestantism are associated historically with the British administration, strengthening and deepening the association between Irish identity and Catholicism.

With much of health care under the control of the Catholic Church, allied to powerful lobbies in medicine, the authority that Rumbold refers to may have been shared between medical science and the Church to a certain degree, but its control over medical ethics and appointments gave the Church a central dominance in health care. Much of the infrastructure, in buildings and land, is Church property, and Catholic bodies, whose control, although diminished, is still evident, particularly in the control of medical ethics concerning reproduction, run many voluntary hospitals.

Forces of change

The drive toward the provision of spiritual care rather than religious care in palliative care and other health care settings has arisen from a number of factors. Rumbold (2002) identifies two key reasons. First, before the 1970s religious care was offered by particular religious groups or denominations, with ministers working as chaplains within hospitals or drawn from local communities. Increasing professionalisation of chaplaincy has led to denominational appointments being superseded by ecumenical chaplaincies. Second, the religious affiliations of patients have become more diverse, and while a majority of people acknowledge some religious connection, this is more commonly stated as Christian rather than denominational;

at the same time the number of people with no religious affiliation has increased (*op. cit*, 5).

Given these changes, chaplains have looked for ways of extending ministry to all people, arguing that only some people are religious but that spirituality is fundamental to all. At the same time as these developments, the hospice movement emerged, incorporating spirituality and spiritual care as a key aspect of the model of care. Rumbold argues (*op. cit.*, 6) that as the first literature on spiritual care came out of this movement, the current wider interest in spiritual care is associated in part with the mainstreaming of hospice care as palliative care.

Walter has stated that a disproportionate number of chaplains in health care are women and that a disproportionate number may also be gay—though quite where the evidence for this assertion comes from is puzzling—and he argues that both these groups are generally kept at arm's length by most churches (2002, 136). Working in health care settings and outside of organised churches gives these chaplains the opportunity to develop personally and theologically more adventurous approaches and to focus on spiritual care rather than religious care.

The factors that Rumbold has documented which have driven the change from religious to spiritual care have not arisen in Ireland. The situation in health care before the 1970s, described by Rumbold, still exists in Ireland. With the vast majority of the population professing to be Catholic, the role for ministers of other faiths is minimal. In large general hospitals it is common for chaplaincy departments to have ordained ministers from Catholic and Anglican traditions, or for ministers from minority faiths to be called as and when the need arises, as was the case in the chaplaincy department in St Theresa's.

Rumbold has identified a fall in the numbers of people affiliated to specific denominations, in addition to a rise in the numbers of people with no religious affiliation. While there has been a rise in the numbers of people professing no religious affiliation in Ireland—the 2006 census shows an increase of 34%—the actual numbers involved are small: a total of 186,318 people have no stated religion; all other religions showed an increase in affiliation, which reverses the position found elsewhere. In addition, there has been a dramatic fall in the numbers of vocations to religious life, as documented in Chapter 2. It would appear that the position in Ireland for the Catholic Church is the reverse of elsewhere; the problem is in providing enough clergy to serve the population, not of finding a large enough population to serve.

A female perspective

Cicely Saunders, in establishing hospice care, emphasised the hospice as a home and the hospice community as a family. Kübler-Ross is not identified specifically with palliative care, but her work on death and dying has been considered by Klass (1981) as playing a symbolic role, by which the public, masculine, rational world of technology could be fought by the female, private, family-related sphere where feelings are the guide to human meaning. This emphasis on home and family reflects a female rather than a male approach to the care of the dying. An association between femaleness and spirituality has been drawn by King (1999), who argues that feminism has led women into a concern with holism and integration, in the form of spiritual feminism. The focus on spiritual rather than religious care in palliative care can be considered a female focus and discourse which reflect an ideological commitment to inclusiveness, although this focus on spirituality has also been driven by organisational and demographic changes, as identified by Rumbold (2002).

The chaplaincy department at St Theresa's consisted of two female religious sisters and one male priest, in addition to ministers from other faiths who were called as and when the need arose. Fr Michael, as an ordained priest, focused, although by no means exclusively, on a sacramental role. By virtue of their sex, this role was not open to Sisters Pauline and Bernadette. From my conversations with these two sisters it was evident that their focus was on the spiritual rather than the religious care of patients and families, and for them spiritual care centred on relationships with people.

Within the Catholic Church the ordination of women is completely outside of practice and beliefs, but the pragmatic need to provide some kind of pastoral care in the face of current limited resources of personnel has led to the opening up of chaplaincy to lay people, including women. Lay people and religious sisters cannot perform a sacramental role and therefore are only able to provide limited religious, as in sacramental, care. A way to develop this role and to extend pastoral care is to emphasise spiritual rather than religious care.

While the predominant discourse within palliative care, certainly in the UK, is spirituality rather than religion, in Ireland there appears to be a dual discourse, one which is male, traditional and focused on a sacramental role—the letter from the Irish bishops which emphasised the role of sacraments in palliative care is an example of this—and another which is female, spiritual and focused on relationship.

Growing Protestantism

There is still a very large percentage of the population whose stated religion is Catholic, although the degree to which this can be ascribed to belief rather than belonging has already been raised. The latest census figures, already discussed, show a small increase in the numbers of people who have no stated religion and an increase of people who are affiliated with a number of Protestant faiths. Some of these increases can be explained by immigration, but this does not account for the total number.

A focus on individualism is characteristic of Protestantism, in which the relationship with God is directly between the individual and God and not mediated through the priest, as is the case in Catholicism. The debate concerning funeral eulogies in 2000, discussed in Chapter 2, can be considered as a sign of increasing individualism within the existing Church structures.

The personalisation of funerary rituals may become an interesting reversal of the Church's elimination of wake amusements, discussed in Chapter 2. While wake amusements died out and the Church control of funerary rituals took hold, this occurred at a time when the power of the Catholic Church was in the ascendant—Inglis (1998) has documented the rise in power of the Catholic Church from the nineteenth to the early to mid-twentieth century. Today, in spite of objections by

Christian churches to eulogies and other features of the personalisation of funerary rituals, in practice these continue to be conducted by family members, at the discretion of the local priest.

Given Taylor's argument (1995), outlined in Chapter 2, that each time a new religious form takes shape it does so with pre-existing materials—language, objects, place and notions—it may be that with an increasing, although slow, shift toward individualism in Irish society new forms of religious practice, focusing on the spiritual and the individual rather than on the religious and the institutional, will take place within the Church rather than outside of the existing structures.

An additional discourse

The earlier (Chapter 2) discussion on the work of Michael Kearney (2000), who advocates the integration of Hippocratic and Asklepian models in a new model of health care, suggests the emergence of another and secular discourse which may fit alongside the religious discourse. The focus on healing, from the Asklepian model, offers a different but parallel view.

The religious discourse offers the Sacrament of the Sick, an anointing with holy oils and the saying of specific prayers, as a mechanism for healing. This sacrament has evolved from the older sacrament of Extreme Unction, which was received by people before they died. The giving of Extreme Unction was governed by strict rules; for instance, it was important that it was administered to the dying person at or extremely close to the moment of death, and Lysaght (1995) has documented occasions when the priest was not informed that death had already occurred as this would have prevented the sacrament being administered. This sacrament has now changed to a more general Sacrament of the Sick, which can be received at any stage of an illness and which seemed to bring considerable consolation to those who received it. This was observed not only by the chaplains in this study but also by the nursing staff. The chaplains spoke about a power that could be accessed through this sacrament, bringing a sense of God's presence with the patient. One of the nursing staff observed that it brought a sense of grace and that people seemed to gain inner peace from it.

Kearney, although writing from a secular perspective, advocates the provision of an environment in which healing can happen. This healing is not brought about by the health care professionals but by the individual; the task of the professionals is to provide a space and environment in which it can happen. In a similar way, while the Sacrament of the Sick is administered by the priest, the grace and inner peace that it brings come from God; the sacrament facilitates a direct connection between the individual and God, according to the Church.

These two approaches, the religious and the secular, operate as twin strands of a discourse on healing, one private and individual and facilitated by health care professionals, and the other religious and facilitated by the priest. These two perspectives run parallel and are not in opposition. Keegan and van Doorslaer (2001) have argued that more than one reference or guide is used in contemporary Ireland; these two parallel and not opposing perspectives suggest that, certainly in some areas, this is the case.

A 'good death'

Bloch and Parry (1982) have argued that a 'good death' is one that suggests 'some level of control over the biological event and is concerned with the restoration of order'. It was clear from Chapter 1 that the context in which death occurs shapes an understanding of a 'good death' and the 'manner of parting'. Aspects of a 'good death' such as peace, acceptance, dealing with 'unfinished business' and achieving resolution can be considered in the context of the restoration of order over the disorder that death brings and serve to 'make the parting as easy and pleasant as possible' (Elias 1985). These aspects have been documented in the historical, folklore and contemporary accounts (Kellehear 1990; Lysaght 1995; Gittings 1999; Morgan 1999, amongst others), as discussed in Chapter 1. Bradbury (1999) clearly showed the degree to which a 'good death' is negotiated and not fixed. In contexts where these aspects cannot be achieved, such as accidental death or when people die sooner than expected, there are attempts to restore order of some kind—the making of some sort of 'good death' in a sense—and a frequent rationale or explanation is one of 'natural' or individual death, in which the person died in a way that reflected their life (*ibid.*).

A 'good death' in palliative care

A 'good death' in palliative care shares characteristics with a 'good death' in other settings and also features aspects of a 'good death' such as dealing with 'unfinished business', resolution, and peace and acceptance. The development of palliative care within cancer care, however, has led to an emphasis on these aspects in ways that are facilitated by the characteristics of the illness, as discussed in Chapter 1. Improved health care, and in particular improvements in the treatment of cancer, makes a prognosis clearer; it also means that many people spend a longer time living with incurable illness. As a result, it can be more difficult to hide the truth about a terminal illness, or at least more difficult to manage non-disclosure. Legislative changes in the US have driven the initial emphasis on communication and open awareness (Field and Copp 1999), alongside other influential work by Glaser and Strauss (1965) on awareness contexts. Allied to this is Saunders's conceptualisation of total pain, facilitated through multi-disciplinary team working (Baines 1990). Together, communication and open awareness and the resolution of multi-dimensional pain can, arguably, lead to an intense focus over what can often be a short period of time under the care of the palliative care services.

A 'good death': the individual and the social

This research has considered a 'good death' as comprising separate but intertwined aspects—an individual aspect and also a social aspect. The individual, while separate, is always part of and related to the social experience of death and dying. Considerable attention was paid by staff, in this study, to the individual aspect of a 'good death'. Understanding and facilitating person-focused care sometimes meant a minimal professional input, such as people dying at home with little or no involvement of the service, or returning a patient to a chaotic home environment which may seem in conflict with patient care but ultimately meets the primary aim.

A central question when considering a 'good death' is whose 'good death' is being talked about. There are clearly a number of social actors involved, and while the primary focus of care is the dying person, the remit of palliative care also includes the family. The social aspects of a 'good death' must also include the professional staff (Dekkers *et al.* 2002). Finding a way to reconcile and manage potentially conflicting perspectives and needs is a challenging and intricate task.

Different perspectives

Differences in perspective between the dying person, family members and the professional staff have been discussed in Chapter 1 (Payne and Langley-Evans 1996; Heaven and Maguire 1997; Kellehear 2001). Payne and Langley-Evans (1996) have suggested that a reason for the disparity may be a different focus: the perspective of staff may aim to maintain the organisational stability of hospice work, and in doing so may constrain patterns of dying. In the Payne and Langley-Evans study patients were found to be more concerned with dying quietly, preferably during sleep, or even dying suddenly, whereas staff were more concerned with a lack of physical pain, the presence of the family and that the patient should show no anxiety. This difference in focus highlights key issues—that of the different aims that may be held by those involved and how potentially conflicting aims may be resolved.

A question of aims

Person-focused care in palliative care has as its primary aim the care of the dying person; at the same time, providing this type of care involves more than one person and more than one perspective. There may be a conflict of aims which can be difficult to resolve. At an extreme end of potential conflicts patients may wish for euthanasia or physician-assisted suicide, which is in direct conflict with the aims of professional staff. Less extreme but just as difficult to resolve are issues concerning patient autonomy, which may conflict with the needs and wishes of family members or the clinical expertise of professional staff. For instance, patients may wish to remain conscious and alert, but in refusing sedative medication they may experience considerable pain and distress, which can be difficult and upsetting for family members and professional staff. Open communication and awareness of death and dying, advocated by palliative care, may be in conflict with the views of the family. This difficulty can be further exacerbated by inter-family conflicts; some family members may want to protect the dying person from knowledge of the terminal illness while others do not. The professional staff may find working with patients and families without an open awareness of the terminal illness difficult and in conflict with the model of care.

Kelner and Bourgeault (1993) have advocated that health professionals should acknowledge patients' autonomy and accommodate their wishes by allowing them more control of the dying trajectory by establishing a partnership in decision-making. Being clear about the aims of the service, i.e. the aim of being person-focused, brings clarity to difficult decision-making, although the issue of patient autonomy is complex and difficult, as was clear from this research.

In order to know the individual aims and preferences it is necessary to engage in a relationship or partnership, as Kelner and Bourgeault (1993) advocate. Relationship of some kind is necessary, certainly in order to understand and facilitate a 'good death', both individually and socially. A 'good death', in this study, was a death that was in harmony with these relationships, relationships which in turn were shaped and influenced by the cultural and social landscape in which they were situated. Throughout the research people in this study spoke frequently about relationship being at the heart of palliative care. If that is the case it raises questions about the nature of the relationship, with whom and where this relationship takes place, and the manner in which it is conducted.

Spiritual care in palliative care

This study has, in addition to an exploration of a 'good death', attempted to reach an understanding of spirituality and spiritual care in palliative care. The previous discussion on the Catholic Church—historically and contemporaneously—has shown that this institution has played a critical role in the creation of a Catholic culture. There is some move toward a discourse on spirituality and a view of people as being primarily spiritual rather than religious, reflecting a shift toward a more individualistic society, and these changes reflect societal changes elsewhere. Nevertheless, some aspects of these changes and the role of religious practice and belief in Ireland show a reversal of trends elsewhere.

A reversal of trends

Ireland still has a very high number of people affiliated to organised religion, especially Catholicism. A shift toward spirituality may, in part, be forced by a reduction in the number of ordained priests able to undertake sacramental duties rather than by a lack of a denominational population. The control by the Church of social institutions, such as education, in the past suggests that in Ireland it may be a case of 'belonging but not necessarily believing', a reversal of that found elsewhere (Davie 2000).

Palliative care promotes an ideal of inclusiveness. Spirituality is considered as a fundamental part of humanity and common to all, whereas religious needs are more specific (Rumbold 2002). It is not surprising, therefore, that spirituality and spiritual care is the dominant discourse of palliative care *(ibid.*, 6). Because spirituality is common to all, and individualistic, it is not possible to come up with a definition that can encapsulate it. 'No pithy definition', according to Kellehear (2002, 169), 'is adequate to capture the diversity and complexity of spiritual desire.' In this study, while people clearly distinguished between religion and spirituality, all attempts at definition were vague; people felt that it was more than religion but were not quite sure how it was more. There was a sense that spirituality was something integral to the individual; it was what is individual about each person and what makes a connection between the individual and the surrounding world, whether or not this encompassed something or someone larger than the individual.

While spirituality and spiritual needs may be hard to define, people do have religious needs, as clearly demonstrated in this study and others, such as Kellehear

1990. Kellehear (2000b) has considered spiritual needs as a desire for transcendence, outlined in Chapter 1, incorporating needs in a number of dimensions that include religion. Kellehear's model in terms of dimensions of need was used as an initial guide to the interview questions in this research. The themes identified by Kellehear (2000b) are reflected in some measure in the aspects of a 'good death' described in Chapter 8. What did emerge strongly in this research, however, was an emphasis on relationships, and the chaplains in this study clearly saw spiritual care as a matter of relationship.

Kellehear has argued that the discussions on spiritual care—in terms of language and preferred storylines—have adopted a rather clinical, acute care style, because 'the emphasis is not on health, normality, culture or community but on crises, problems, professional territory or rivalry' (2002, 169). This emphasis is missing in Ireland; this may have to do with the factors already outlined, especially as a culture of Catholicism renders it much easier for all staff, and not just chaplains, to talk about spirituality and sometimes religious needs and questions. The absence of the professional rivalry about who can or cannot deliver spiritual care which has appeared in much of the, largely UK, palliative and nursing literature outlined in Chapter 1 may be due to the 'naturalness' of religion that has already been discussed.

A community connection

Kellehear (2002) has argued that a desire for transcendence has situational, moral, biographical and religious sources. He states that in each of these areas there is a need for community connection and for social action rather than simple discussion with health professionals (*op. cit.*, 170). While acknowledging that there is an important role for listening, discussion, counselling and joint reflection with professionals, he suggests that the major role lies with the person with the terminal illness, with his or her self and with his or her usual social world (*op. cit.*, 170). Spiritual needs therefore have a large community-based component, with friends and family. The person with the terminal illness is, Kellehear argues, the main social actor, who needs to act, and that action needs to take place within the patient's own community (*op. cit.,* 171). This view of spiritual needs and how they can be addressed also involves relationship—relationship between the terminally ill patient and his or her social world, which includes, but is not restricted to, the palliative care service and professionals.

If relationship is involved in spiritual care and also in facilitating person-focused palliative care, then palliative care is, in a sense, spiritual care. Spirituality is common to all and can mean 'whatever is sacred to people'; this does not necessarily have to be religious, but spiritual care, when embodied in authentic relationship, can touch what is sacred. If relationship is central in spiritual care and central in facilitating person-focused palliative care, then relationship is at the heart of palliative care, and this again raises the same questions: what is the nature of the relationship, with whom and where does it take place, and in what manner is it conducted?

Summary

It has been argued that contemporary Ireland is now characterised by a changing landscape in which more than one reference or guide is used. The demographic changes show the signs of an emerging diversity; tensions between the individual and the institutional churches, demonstrated in the debate on funeral eulogies and the development of another, and secular, discourse on healing, are signs of this shift. A central question remains—whether this emergent individualism and associated discourse will have equal access and equal weight.

This chapter has examined the three aspects that the research set out to explore: understandings of a 'good death', the spiritual care dimension of palliative care, and the influences of culture. This analysis has shown that relationship is at the heart of palliative care but this relationship is one that has been shaped by the social and historical context. The legacy of the past, which includes the complex relationship between influential groups within the Catholic Church and the medical profession in the development of an inequitable health service and the role of the Catholic Church in the creation of a culture of Catholicism, has formed the basis of present-day relationships and the language through which these are conducted. The nature of these relationships, and with whom and the manner in which they are conducted, is the focus of the following and final chapter.

CHAPTER 10

The angle of repose: finding the point of balance

Introduction

Small (2003) has considered the issue of user involvement in palliative care in a discussion on the future of the NHS. He states that the user involvement project is 'fundamentally about how to reconcile the existence of institutional and professional agendas' which have built up over time in the context of service planning and delivery and the agenda built 'out of the subjective, embodied experience of caring for someone who is ill' (2003, 20). The relationship between these two agendas also needs to be examined in an Irish context. Just as in the previous chapter the structural relationship in Ireland was seen to consist of the health service, the palliative care service and the Catholic Church, the relationships under examination in this chapter reflect this additional dimension.

This chapter explores the nature of this relationship, how and with whom it is conducted, the dynamics involved and the terms of negotiation. The conceptual framework of cartography, applied from the outset of the research, has served to make more explicit differences in the relationships dependent upon location of care. The angle of repose, which is the title of this chapter, is the point at which separate lines intersect and support one another; a number of lines can be placed together at this angle of repose to form a supporting arch. In this discussion, these lines can be considered as the relationships between the social actors, the social institutions and the context in which they are situated. The focus of the following discussion is the way in which they meet and support each other—or not, as the case may be.

Relationships in palliative care

Relationship is at the heart of palliative care, but who is this relationship with and how is it conducted? Relationships in health care often focus on those between the patient and health care professionals, in terms of lay and professional perspectives. The term 'health care professionals' can, however, disguise the fact that in practice this means a lot of people, especially within the multi-disciplinary team working of the palliative care model. Similarly, the term 'lay' disguises the fact that a patient lives within his or her family, friends and wider community, as Kellehear (2000) has argued.

A complex weave

Deckers *et al*. (2002) have argued for the inclusion of the perspective of professional staff in understandings of a 'good death', and Small (2003) makes explicit the agenda of the organisation and service. The palliative care service, the organisation, the professional and other staff working within the organisation, other patients and their family members, the community, friends, family members and the individual who is dying all have a place in the social dimension. Earlier discussions have focused on the influence of the Catholic Church in developing and shaping health care institutions and social and cultural practices in Ireland, so this bedrock of influence must also be borne in mind. The multi-disciplinary model of palliative care increases the potential number of professional staff engaged in a relationship with the patient and the family members. The often large numbers of family members frequently referred to in this study increase the number of interactions with the patient and the complexities of these relationships. So it would appear that the social world of the dying person can be a very crowded place, and consequently the social aspect of a 'good death' is a complex weave of interactions.

A figurational approach

The grouping together of social actors under two headings—a lay and a professional perspective—disguises complex interactions and that these perspectives are informed by sometimes conflicting sets of information, knowledge and beliefs. The perspective of professionals is shaped and informed by specific technical knowledge, expertise and experience. The social actors incorporated within the lay perspectives also have their own previous experience of health care professionals and medical science. Not all of these experiences have been positive and people may feel let down by the medical system; Sontag (1989) suggests that the promises of medical science are not consistent with people's experience. The lay view of health and illness, without a professional background, tends to be broad-ranging and multi-causal; Murray and McMillan (1993) have reported that older people are more likely to attribute the cause of cancer to factors such as luck or chance. Williams and Popay (1994, 123) argue that lay knowledge about health and illness is subjective but highly coherent. Social class (Pill and Stott 1982), age (Blaxter and Paterson 1982) and gender (Blaxter 1990) are also factors that influence lay concepts of health and illness.

Elias's (1987) 'figurational' or 'sociogenetic' approach offers a way of understanding the patterns of social interaction and interdependence between people, groups and societies that encompass every form of cooperation and conflict and which are rarely static and unchanging (Mennell 1996, 15).

Elias has considered the social processes at work in long-term social development and believes that the stage of development attained by society can be identified and measured in relation to a 'triad of basic controls' (Elias 1978, 156–7). These controls are firstly the extent of society's capacity to exert control over non-human forces and events or 'forces of nature'; secondly the extent of its control over interpersonal relationships and events or 'social forces'; and thirdly the extent to which each of the members of a society has control over him or herself as an individual (Mennell 1992). These three types of control develop and function in interdependence with each other and with the development of knowledge, but Elias contends that this interdependence is not to be understood as simple parallel increases of three types in step with each other. Rather these controls interact with each other in a more paradoxical way; as the capacity for taking a more detached view and control over natural forces increases, this tends to increase the difficulties in extending control over social relationships and the feelings in thinking about them (*ibid.*, 169).

Elias (1987) argues that when people are in positions of vulnerability and insecurity it is more difficult to control strong feelings about events that deeply affect their lives, and more difficult to approach those events with detachment as long as they have little ability to control the course of events. On the other hand, Elias argues, it is also difficult to extend understanding and control of these events if they are not approached with a greater detachment. This produces a kind of double bind that can obstruct the growth of knowledge in respect of all three levels of the triad—the 'always interconnected levels of the technological, the social and the psychological'. The interconnection between the three levels may serve not only to impede growth of knowledge but also to put the process into reverse gear (Mennell 1992, 170). While impediments and reversals of change occur, over the very long term these social processes produce developmental change of and within societies and individuals.

Elias (1985, 28) has stated that 'dying is at present a largely unformed situation, a blank area on the social map', as discussed in earlier chapters; this study, in its exploratory approach, has attempted to fill in some of these blank areas. Using Elias's figurational approach to consider the development of palliative care, the more holistic approach to the care of the dying can be seen in terms of a continuum of social development in very broad terms.

The developmental processes involved in the emergence of palliative care and the key aspects of communication and open awareness, for instance, illustrate the different stages of development at each of the three levels suggested by Elias: the technological—developments in cancer care which, as already stated, mean that more people are living longer with cancer and therefore full disclosure of the prognosis becomes necessary; the social—the development of palliative care as a model of care that manages the social relationship between the increasing technological information and expertise and the disclosure and mechanism of living with that information; and the psychological—the individual response to the implications of that information. Difficulties between professionals working in the health care services who do not have the same level of commitment to open awareness and communication and palliative care, and the health care services

(Young and Cullen 1996, 112) and the shift from full to conditional awareness (Field and Copp 1999) demonstrate that these stages do not necessarily work smoothly with each other and illustrate the kind of 'double bind' referred to by Elias.

Power relations

Increasing medicalisation, informed by an ever-increasing technical knowledge of the body, has tended to polarise lay and professional perspectives, a polarisation that is made explicit in the work of Foucault and his conceptualisation of the 'clinical gaze' (1976). Foucault argues that the patient is constructed under the 'clinical gaze' of the physician and reduced to the pathologies displayed. He makes explicit the dynamics of interaction, for example in his conceptualisation of surveillance and resistance; however, this conceptualisation assumes that these perspectives are in opposition to each other. Viewed differently, what can be considered as surveillance from a lay perspective can be considered as observation from a medical one; observation has been a valuable tool in increasing medical knowledge, which in turn has improved the quality of life of people who are ill. While there is no doubt that within the interaction between these two perspectives there is a dynamic of power, the balance of which can at times be very unequal, this dynamic can be observed in any relationship between groups or people who are bonded together through interdependence on each other (Mennell 1996).

Nettleton (1995, 157) has stated that there is an inherent paradox in the critique of medicalisation—if medicine takes the social aspects of health and illness into account it is accused of medical imperialism; if it does not it is accused of medical reductionism. This is really a case of 'damned if you do and damned if you don't'. The incorporation of social aspects of health and illness and a shift toward a more holistic view of people and health care are embodied within the development of the hospice movement and palliative care. Foucault's later (1982) development of 'pastoral power' also offers a way to consider the interaction within holism in modern medicine, and especially in palliative care. Pastoral power is a form of surveillance, according to Foucault, that directs its gaze inward toward people as individual subjects rather than as objects, and which implies knowledge of the consciousness and an ability to direct it (Foucault 1982, 214). McGowen (1994) has suggested that in the conjoining of these two words the traditional pastoral concerns of the clergy have become generalised and redirected toward health and well-being. As previously stated, within any relationship between groups or people who are interdependent there is a dynamic of power that can at times be very unequal but at other times more evenly balanced (Mennell 1996). Although the model of palliative care has at its centre a holistic view of patients and families and adopts a person-centred approach to care, this does not necessarily ensure that the balance of power within the relationships between patients and family members and professional staff is always an equal one.

Foucault's conceptualisations make explicit the inherent dynamics present within relationships. Mennell (1992, 170) states that as societies become more complex, increasing numbers of people become more interdependent. The result is longer chains and denser webs of interaction. In this study, these longer chains and webs of interaction were apparent between the health service, the religious order and the Catholic Church, the palliative care community, and the patient and the family, who in turn have chains and webs of interaction between their own wider community and the palliative care and other health care services.

Webs of interaction

Kellehear (2002) has considered the terminally ill patient as situated within a wider community of relatives and friends. This community may share a similar set of beliefs and values, in a sense a community culture. Small (1993, 73) has suggested that there are difficulties associated with a community action model for health education, such as a lack of a direct common concern. Yet it is precisely the potential lack of common concerns that may be made visible by considering the views expressed in this study as reflective of communities and their cultural beliefs and values rather than as lay and professional perspectives. It may also show more clearly the chains and webs of interaction that Elias has referred to. The professional and other staff working in palliative care organisations share a similar set of beliefs and values—an organisational culture that was evident from Chapter 4. There are other 'communities' which are linked, such as that of the health service—a contrast between the values of the health service in general settings was also evident. The religious community involved in the palliative care organisation in this study is also part of a wider religious community and the community of the Catholic Church.

Cultures in focus: the Irish health service and palliative care

The palliative care services were perceived very positively in contrast to the general health service in Ireland. For professional staff who had worked in other settings, the organisational focus on care was a major motivating factor for working in palliative care, in addition to the supportive environment and the team working aspect of the model.

Bradshaw (1996b) has stated that nursing has rediscovered its theological and pastoral base, and for some of the nursing staff the focus on caring for dying people was a key attraction and reflected their own spiritual perspective and personal values. For other nurses, however, the motivation for working in palliative care was less about caring for dying people and more about a good working environment in which there was a much higher ratio of nursing staff to patients. The person-focused approach of palliative care is facilitated by the high nursing staff to patient ratio and, according to one of the doctors in the study, palliative care was protected from staff cutbacks, unlike other parts of the health service. This level of staffing facilitates the caring aspects of nursing, and protection from staff cutbacks facilitates that level of attention to patients and family members.

The organisational values described in Chapter 4 demonstrated that the person-focused approach of palliative care also included the professional staff. Formal and informal support was provided, particularly for the nursing staff, and understanding was demonstrated when family and personal difficulties occurred. This level of care for staff seemed to have a knock-on positive impact, increasing commitment and positive perceptions—hallmarks, in fact, of any mutually supportive relationship. This appears as a potentially ever-expanding positive organisational model, in contrast to comments made by staff about other health care environments in which poor staffing levels and pressure of work clearly decreased levels of commitment and increased levels of frustration.

The positive perception of the palliative care services expressed by many of the people in this study can also be understood in the context of general health care services in Ireland, which have been shown to be inequitable and subject to influence from powerful lobbies. The ideological commitment of the organisation to an equitable service, in contrast to other palliative care organisations where patients with private health insurance are facilitated, was a motivating factor for joining the organisation stated explicitly by one member of the professional staff and perceived very positively by staff generally.

In this study some of the staff in the hospice talked to me from the perspective of family members. Many of their comments focused on their very negative experience in other health care settings, and they expressed tremendous gratitude for the care they and their relative received from the palliative care services. For one of the home care nurses it was the palliative care received by her dying father that prompted her own move to train and work in the service. Her comments echo others, such as that it was not the big things like pain and symptom management that counted, although these were also important, but the small details of care like names being remembered and a doilie on the tea tray.

Family members talked about respect and dignity being restored by the palliative care service in contrast to the very poor experiences in general health care settings. A recent study, 'An exploration of dignity in palliative care' (Duarte Enes 2003), explored this concept with patients, relatives and professionals in palliative care and found that a lack of resources and poor organisation eroded dignity. A lack of time on the part of professional staff made patients feel a nuisance and undermined their feelings of self-worth. Other themes on the meaning of dignity emerged—relationship and belonging, which included being heard and understood, giving and receiving love and being included. Having control of decisions and of what is happening was also considered important, in addition to independence, space and privacy (*ibid.*, 264). These aspects of caring for patients are facilitated by the person-focused approach of palliative care and more difficult to achieve in an overworked and understaffed health care service.

The culture of palliative care: a closer look

Palliative care as person-focused care marks a departure from general health care, which is focused on cure and features a more task-orientated approach. Nevertheless, palliative care is still health care and offers opportunities for professional staff to engage more fully with the patient, family members and other professionals. As such, it is potentially more rewarding for staff, although not all patients and family members may wish to have this level of engagement.

Biswas (1993) has argued that the creation of a medical specialism of palliative medicine effectively means that doctors are motivated by career opportunities to expand their focus from pain control to symptom control and their concern from the final few days and weeks to the long-term relief of pain and symptoms. Kearney (1992) has also expressed concerns that the drive to research symptomatology in order to maintain the specialism's status focuses on a narrow medical field in palliative care.

In this study doctors spoke, in relation to team working, about the value of the perspective of other professions, such as social work, as well as the expansion of their own role as one of relationship with patients and families. Nurses, too, appreciated working within a team model, although some expressed the view that the traditional hierarchical professional positions of doctors and nurses were still in place, which mirrors the view expressed by a non-medical team member at St Christopher's Hospice (Walter 1994, 165). The multi-disciplinary model has evolved in many palliative care settings to an interdisciplinary model. According to Abu-Saad (2001), the goal of interdisciplinary palliative care is the provision of excellent care taking into consideration the complexity of care provided, the utilisation of the appropriate skills provided by team members and the minimisation of fragmentation of care. Coyle (1997) has identified a number of barriers to the implementation of collaborative palliative care services: the culture of the institution, such as the hierarchical authority of the physician in relation to the nurse, issues regarding 'ownership of the patient', and the question of expertise with regard to profession, service and team.

The comments made by some of the nurses in this study reflect a concern about the level and nature of involvement with patients and family members. Several nurses were not happy with questioning patients about their concerns: 'I don't like this gut stuff, you know, digging in and trying to find out what is in there. Because you could open a can of worms with someone who is vulnerable and near death anyway and I am not into that much'.

Some nurses expressed concern at the amount of personal information that was discussed at meetings—'Sometimes I say to myself if this was me and my family, how would I feel?' While being in receipt of considerable amounts of intimate information about people was accepted as part of their professional job, one nurse was also concerned about the level of professionalism amongst care assistants who could be '*working in a supermarket one week and then at a psychosocial meeting the next week*'. This nurse was also concerned about the level of professionalism in conversations between family members and care assistants. While reservations were expressed about some aspects of the care assistant's role, care assistants may see their role as taking on some of the observational tasks of nursing; one of the care assistants felt that it was part of her job to surreptitiously observe patients—'You might just sit and you are letting on that you are just sitting there and you are there watching them'.

Professional staff enjoyed the expanded role that palliative care offers, although some staff, doctors and social workers in particular, met with resistance from some family members and patients. Resistance to the new holistic model of care was countered by a return to a more traditional role such as using the authority of doctors— 'A lot of [patients] would listen to the doctor rather than the non-medical staff. You have to ask the doctor to say it because then they will say "the doctor said".'

Patients and family members may also resist the additional service that palliative care offers; one family member only wanted to see doctors:—'He steadfastly refused to be involved with anyone other than doctors. In fact he used the words "keep those social workers and counsellors away from me"'.

The home care nurses frequently spoke of resistance to the involvement of the social worker and felt that there was a problematic perception of the role of the social worker. The resistance in one instance resulted in a more 'gentle' approach and a strategy whereby the chaplain was suggested in order to start the patient talking:

> *'maybe we'll go gently and maybe if they go and see the chaplain they will get used to talking but maybe then the social worker might come in later on and there might be a way of getting around that'.*

The social workers that I spoke with were clear that involvement with that aspect of the service was a choice; however, if patients and family members 'failed to engage' with the 'opportunity to address issues…then the patient may die without any of that work being done'. Seeing death and dying as an opportunity is part of the ideology of palliative care and part of that culture's beliefs and values, but it may not be a view that others share.

Invisible work

The palliative care community also includes those who work in the organisation in a variety of roles. In this study I spoke with administrative and kitchen staff and volunteers. Some of the administrative staff had prior experience of the palliative care services in relation to their own relatives, and their sense of commitment to the service and the organisation was considerable. Their appreciation of the values of the organisation was clear, especially in relation to equity of service. Many staff members managed aspects of patient and staff care that were not necessarily apparent or visible to professional staff. The care taken in the selection of menus in the canteen so that nursing staff could more fully appreciate a break from their work was just one example. Another might be the response to the genuine distress of a telephone caller to the hospice although 'bereavement support' was not part of the job description.

Hoad's (1991) study on volunteers in the independent hospice movement has highlighted the difficulties of boundaries between volunteers and paid staff, which appear to be unclear and can lead to considerable tension between staff and volunteers. These types of difficulties did not arise in relation to volunteers in this study, but a similar uncertainty about boundaries was apparent amongst some of the administrative staff, who felt that 'there is a certain line you can't cross'. Some of the staff felt that in doing their work they were indirectly looking after patients, even though they might not be in positions where any direct contact was necessary. In one instance reported to me, however, a patient chose a member of the administration staff to talk with, rather than the professional staff. In cases where some contact was part of the job, there was sometimes uncertainty about their role, as they were 'not the professionals'. At around the time my research began, some level of support was put in place for administration staff. The chaplaincy department provided this—a development initiated by administration staff. The type of work undertaken by administration and other staff and volunteers in the hospice is akin to the type of necessary but often invisible work that is undertaken in any social group. It was clear that these staff members and volunteers were highly committed to the values and beliefs of the palliative culture and organisation and undertook considerable responsibility for maintaining and enacting these values, although much of this work may not be visible.

The locus of control

Examining the relationships between professional staff and patients and family members according to location of care has made explicit differences between the communities. Saunders (1965) has described the community at St Christopher's

Hospice as 'the kind of family and home that can give the kind of welcome and hospitality of a good home'. The ideal of the hospice movement was to provide a form of extended family which sought to give patients a more personal form of care and stressed the importance of including the family as well as the dying person within the remit of care, as already discussed in Chapter 1. Nevertheless, this presentation of hospice as home is selective (Froggatt 1997). Froggatt argues that negative aspects of family life, such as tensions and disagreements, are not part of the home-like atmosphere promoted by hospices. The examination of relationship according to location of care clearly showed that home is the locus of control, and which home the relationship takes place in influences the balance of the relationship.

Visitors and occupiers

Palliative care professionals frequently spoke about being visitors in the home of the patients and some of the staff clearly loved this position, describing it as a privilege. But being a visitor entailed fitting in with the prevailing culture of the family—'it's their home, it's not yours, so you go in as a professional to offer services but you have to be respectful of people's views and wishes and you have to go around things gently'.

Conflicts over key issues in palliative care, such as open awareness and communication, caused some of the professional staff considerable difficulty, however. Professionals spoke about the culture of the family which sometimes fitted with the culture of palliative care: 'the family that can talk about things openly and where things are open and above board would seem to us to be better'. A matching culture certainly made the job of the professionals much easier; the description in Chapter 6 of 'edging through the door' in some houses cannot make the job easy for any person, and clearly within the home care teams there was considerable and ongoing debate about working with patients and families who were not aware or open about the terminal illness. Some of the professional staff took the view that their job was to work with the existing pattern of communication within the family and to leave this intact. This involved working with patients and families to help them deal more fully with what is happening but not to cause disruption to a family pattern that has existed for a long time and which will still be there when the involvement of the palliative care services ceased:

> *'at the end of the day leave them intact because they have had this pattern for so long, after we are gone, they will still be there, they still have to relate. The remaining members of the family still have to relate'.*

The role of the home care nurses, viewed as providing appropriate support and facilitating the family in caring for the terminally ill person, was seen as challenging but potentially very satisfying for many of those I spoke with. A large part of the support provided by palliative care teams for patients and families at home was, in addition to pain and symptom management, a focus on practical aspects of help. One home care nurse related how being able to provide a special bed downstairs in the family home and encouraging the family to draw up a rota of friends to provide some additional support had enabled the family to continue caring for their family member at home.

This focus on the value of practical assistance was also reflected in the views of terminally ill patients in a study conducted by Raynes *et al.* (2000) in which all respondents identified their families as a major source of help but also welcomed the visits of home care nurses, financial help with housework and maintenance of their standard of living. Advice and information about what happens after chemotherapy and available financial benefits were also welcomed.

A wider community

The palliative care home care team provide support for the patient and family at home but they may not be the only support that is available. Support for the terminally ill patients and their family members was also present in the wider community of neighbours and friends; the vivid description by one of the home care doctors in this study who sensed a whole community of neighbours protecting and looking after a young dying woman is one example of the wider community that may be part of the patient's social world. In an exploratory study of the role of friends and neighbours in providing support for older people, Nocon and Pearson (2000) found that the role of non-kin carers can be significant in supporting older people in their own homes. One of the main forms of direct support related to older people's quality of life, at a broader level than the support provided by statutory services.

Another aspect of a wider community may be the presence of deceased relatives. Patients and family members may experience the presence and support of deceased relatives, as discussed in Chapter 8, as part of a continuum of relationships that people perceive. Seeing deceased relatives close to death was a frequent experience, frequent enough for one doctor to remark — 'if somebody is seeing dead relatives like they are, I assume they are fairly close [to death]'.

These experiences have also been documented in the general literature (Zaleski 1987; Basford 1990) and some nursing, generally American, literature (Papowitz 1986; Schoenbeck 1993). In the Payne and Langley-Evans (1996) study, already discussed, deathbed visions were referred to by some of the patients but not by staff; the authors note that most people found them reassuring (*op. cit.*, 310). Within the palliative care literature only one study (Barbato *et al.* 1999) has specifically considered the parapsychological phenomena near the time of death and during bereavement, finding them present both as deathbed visions and as 'sense of presence' experiences in bereavement. The authors suggest that possible reasons for the lack of coverage of these experiences in the palliative care literature include a lack of awareness of these phenomena or an unwillingness to speak about them. They also suggest that the mainstream palliative care journals may consider this topic to be 'somewhat "fringy" and are reluctant to publish material that does not meet tight scientific or rational guidelines' (*op. cit.*, 35). The authors further suggest that, as these are common and frequent experiences, it is part of the professional role of palliative care workers to normalise these experiences and to encourage patients and relatives to talk about any unusual event that occurs.

One home care nurse related how, after completing her palliative care course, she visited her terminally ill aunt to 'help her and get her to come to terms with her dying', only to find that her aunt was already having conversations with her dead twin and other sisters. As this nurse was a relative, her aunt may have been more willing to talk about these experiences with her. Many people may not speak of these experiences to professionals for fear of being considered a little strange.

A parallel can be drawn with the 'sense of presence' experiences of many bereaved people and which now form part of the professional bereavement discourse, such as *Continuing bonds* (Klass *et al.* 1996). An early study, 'The hallucinations of widowhood' (Rees 1971), documented these experiences amongst widows in the Welsh/English border area. Rees's study, which arose from research for his MD thesis on mortality rates of the recently bereaved, found that almost half of the widows in his study had hallucinatory or paranormal experiences but that it was unusual for these experiences to be disclosed, even to close friends and relatives, because of a fear that they would be laughed at or considered mad (Rees 1971, 20). Accounts of these experiences have also appeared within sociology (Howarth 1998b; Hallam *et al.* 1999) in a discussion of these experiences as the extension of the social beyond biological death. They are also present in the folklore record (Bennett 1987); Hufford (1982), an American folklorist, has concentrated on the phenomenology of these experiences and suggests that traditional beliefs, such as a belief in ghosts, have emerged to explain the strange experiences we do have, rather than the more usual view that these beliefs determine the nature of the strange experiences we may have.

In a cross-cultural study of deathbed observations by physicians and nurses (Osis and Haraldsson 1977) in North America and northern India, the research found that while deathbed visions were common there were cultural differences; the identity of the visions varied greatly between the two groups in India and the USA. American patients mainly saw deceased persons, while Indian patients predominantly saw religious figures. Lundahl (1982) has argued that the medical observers in this study may have reported what they believed they were supposed to, according to cultural norms, and left out what went against the grain of a particular culture.

Within the Catholic Church, apparitions of saints, the Virgin Mary or other religious figures are known. In the pilot studies conducted for this research some people reported their relative seeing deceased relatives, while others reported their relative seeing, in one instance, the Virgin Mary; this vision was understood as being appropriate to the dying person, who 'had a great devotion to the Virgin Mary'. Within the culture of Catholicism in Ireland it may be that visions of religious figures are common, although there is, as yet, little discussion or research about these experiences.

Changing positions

The in-patient unit in the hospice can be considered to be the home of the professional staff and at the heart of the culture of palliative care. Payne and Langley-Evans (1996) have argued that staff may work to maintain the organisational stability of hospice work and in doing so may constrain patterns of dying. Nevertheless, the hospice as a place is a health care setting and the organisation is a health care organisation with its own set of aims and values, and as such there are, in addition to patient and family needs, staff and organisational needs to be considered.

The resistance to the expanded role of doctors and the interventions of social workers has already been discussed. Nurses play a central role in patient care, and particularly so in the in-patient unit, where they are a constant presence, unlike other professional staff. Hewison has argued that nurses, because of their role, are the 'appointed' arbiters of interactional power in the clinical setting and use persuasion to ensure that patients fall in with their 'understanding of appropriate behaviour' (1995, 79). May (1991) has observed that the structure and process in the organisation of nursing work exert a powerful influence over the types of relationships and communication shared by patients and nurses.

An assumption that lay people lack influence in their interaction with health care workers has been the foundation of research concerning lay–professional interaction (May *et al.* 2001). Early research, such as the ethnographic study of the relationship between nurses, patients and their families in acute wards in a Canadian hospital (Rosenthal *et al.* 1980), found that nurses sought to control the conditions of their work while patients and their families sought to control the conditions of their hospital experience. Rosenthal *et al.* argue that in order to control family members nurses place them into one of three roles—patient, visitor or worker—all of which have implications for nurses' control and authority.

A study in the UK (Allen 2000) suggests that informal carers pose a challenge to the fundamental social organisation of work, and nurses found it hard to involve carers in ways that did not undermine their professional identities and their abilities to deal with the practical aspects of their work. Allen argues that negotiations between formal and informal carers can take place against a highly charged emotional backdrop which may increase difficulties.

Hewison (1995) has argued that nurses exert considerable power over patients and do so through their use of language, by creating most of the verbal communication and controlling the content of the interaction. This power is reinforced in a number of ways; for example, the interactions can resemble those of a parent and child, as demonstrated by the widespread use of 'terms of endearment' such as 'sweetie' and 'darling' (*op. cit.*, 80). The May *et al.* (2001) study has examined the relationship between informal carers and health care workers and has found that both parties act as gatekeepers to the patient and that negotiation was enacted through everyday conversation. The discussion in the previous chapter concerning the cultural language of prayer clearly showed that prayers are one mechanism of communication through which nurses manage patients and family members.

Current research into the power relations between nurses, patients and informal carers has taken place in general health care settings. However, while palliative care is health care it is a different model and more person-focused, which may alter the balance of these relationships.

The hospice as home

As already stated, part of the initial ideology of the hospice movement was to provide a kind of extended family and home for dying people and their families. It was clear that considerable effort was expended to make St Theresa's Hospice as home-like as possible, with attention paid to the furniture, furnishings and the type of food on offer, as discussed in Chapter 6. The involvement of religious orders in health care and in the hospice has left its mark, and although considerable efforts were made to ensure that the hospice was not an overtly Catholic place, it clearly was so and this may not suit all patients, although little real choice exists. Two members of the chaplaincy department were an almost constant presence in the in-patient unit—a presence, it must be said, that seemed welcome to many people, although it is difficult to know to what extent this is really the case. This study did not consider the views of patients about this aspect of care, but given the culture of Catholicism and the suggestion that there may be 'belonging but not necessarily believing', as discussed in the previous chapter, it is difficult to unravel cultural practices from specific religious needs and beliefs.

Most people state a preference to die at home. A prospective study of preferred versus actual place of death among patients referred to a palliative care home care service in Ireland (Tiernan *et al*. 2002) found that 82% of patients expressed a preference to die at home, with a further 11% choosing the hospice, 3% hospital and 3% a nursing home. Fifty-two per cent of the patients in the study died in either a hospice or an acute hospital. The reasons for admission were varied, although the study did find that if extra nursing care had been available more patients would have stayed at home. Forty-two per cent of patients were admitted to either a hospice or hospital because their next of kin were no longer able to cope, 30% were admitted because of intractable symptoms, 8% were admitted because they lived alone although otherwise there was no acute problem, 3% were admitted because of fear of an acute major bleed, 5% were admitted for respite care and their condition deteriorated unexpectedly, and the reason for admission was unknown for a further 12% of the patients (*ibid*., 233).

These figures reflect the findings of this research in which the home care nurses talked about a variety of reasons for admission to the in-patient unit, and carer burden was one of the main reasons in addition to difficult symptom management, as the Tiernan *et al.* study indicates. It was also clear from this study that the reasons for admission were individualistic. Some patients expressed a wish, according to the staff, to avail of the religious and spiritual care at the hospice, others found constant visitors difficult to manage at home, some carers found the intimate tasks involved in caring for their relative difficult, and some people were uncomfortable about death taking place at home.

Caring for patients and family members, some of whom may wish to be in the hospice and others not, can be a difficult task for staff. Although considerable effort was spent in making the hospice appear home-like, the hospice is not the home of the patient and the family, and this position was clearly identified by one of the nurses in the study who described the in-patient unit as 'our territory'. According to this nurse, patients were disempowered in coming into the in-patient unit, visible to her in seeing patients in their pyjamas all day, which would not be the case in their own home, and in staff 'dishing out tablets', which again in the patient's own home they were able to manage themselves.

In an article on proposed voluntary euthanasia legislation in the Isle of Man (*Sunday Times*, 10 August 2003), comments by a retired clinical psychologist living in the Isle of Man, Dr Jeff Garland, suggest that for some people palliative care is not a positive experience:

> *'palliative care is a pretty rocky road—you have to swallow along with your medication, a good deal of well-intentioned reassurance, people trying to play amateur psychologist with you. It's done with the best will in the world, but it can be excruciatingly painful...'.*

In this study one nurse commented on the resistance to persistent questioning made by patients—'if one more person asks me that question'. Positive comments about palliative care by family members in this study were about the small details of care, such as remembering people's names, and the attention to the family, not necessarily about open awareness or family meetings; these comments seemed to echo those of

Saunders (1988) in relation to spiritual care, which she considered often to be in the practical things such as the physical caring for people and paying attention to the family.

Managing a 'good death'

This study has considered a 'good death' as having both an individual and a social dimension. Nurses considered it important to get to know patients before they died; it was satisfying for the staff and helped them to facilitate the individual aspect of a 'good death'. The unravelling and understanding of individual needs and desires were considered to be as important as the control of pain and symptoms. Preferences for the family being present and involved or not, dying in the in-patient unit or at home, and having the involvement of the chaplain or no involvement with this part of the service were seen as individual choices and were accommodated where possible.

The individual nature of each death, also expressed as 'die as you live', was an explanation that was used both when things went according to an idealised version of a 'good death' and when they didn't. So on the one hand, a person dying peacefully and in full acceptance of impending death and in the presence of his family was seen in one instance as reflecting the life that had been lived—a 'good life'. On the other hand, a man dying by himself, without his son being present, which is not part of an idealised version of a 'good death', was explained and understood as an appropriate death given the private nature of the individual and his distant relationship with his son.

Sometimes facilitating the individual needs and desires of patients caused difficulties for staff; for instance, several of the staff mentioned the patient who wanted to die in the chair, and the staff clearly struggled with this—it seemed to make them uncomfortable, as it conflicted with idealised views of a 'good death'. This difficulty highlights the tension between the individual and social dimensions of death. Pauline, one of the chaplains, acknowledged that the need to make it 'the best it can be' is because this makes it easier for other people, such as the family and professional staff.

As Taylor (1989) has stated, death is a potent time for important issues in a culture to be made visible, and the interfaces, and power relations, between the different communities that encompass the social dimension of death become more visible at the period of time close to death. These communities, incorporating the dying person and their relatives and friends, other patients and their families, professional staff and the organisation, have their own needs, which may at times be in conflict. The dying process and the social relationships were clearly managed, as discussed in Chapter 6, and managed by nurses. A 'good death', whether at home or in the hospice, is a death in which all of these relationships are in harmony with each other.

The language used by nursing staff was considered by Hewison (1995) and May *et al.* (2001) as a critical means by which the relationship between patients, family members and staff is negotiated and conducted. In this study, the management strategies in the in-patient unit, and occasionally at home, close to the time of death often included prayers, as discussed in the previous chapter. While prayers and religious rituals at this time seemed important and appropriate for many people, they are also a culturally appropriate and understandable language for some of the communities present and may facilitate harmonisation.

The manner of engagement

This chapter has examined the relationship that is considered to be at the heart of palliative care. It has shown that relationships exist between a myriad of social actors who reside and work within their own cultural communities, which may share some beliefs and values but which may also, at times, be in opposition to each other. While much of the literature on the relationships between patients and health care workers has tended to consider the relationship as an unequal one, this literature has focused on general health care settings. Palliative care is health care but it is a different type of health care, one that is focused on the person, including the family, and aims to provide holistic care. Lay and health communities can be considered to be somewhat in opposition to each other, in the way that Foucault (1976) has made explicit these opposing perspectives. Palliative care, however, positions itself closer to the patient and the family—a midway point of balance between these communities—and the manner of engagement may be characterised as one of negotiation and accommodation, not just on the part of the professional staff and the organisation but also on the part of the patients and family members.

A balancing act

The analysis of the day care service at St Theresa's Hospice showed clearly that the service acted as an in-between space for the organisation, the professional staff and patients and family members. Much of the work of the professional staff was aimed at trying to achieve a balance between resources, the service and the needs of the patients. It is not only in the day care service that the attempt to achieve a balance was evident. An effort to achieve a balance between a home-like environment and the organisational needs was also clear. Getting the balance right between being a supportive organisation and one that functions to support its staff was another challenge.

Drawing fine lines

The person-focused approach of palliative care is a welcome initiative and development within health care but, as Small has argued, there is a need to 'reconcile the existence of institutional and professional agendas' which have built up over time in the context of service planning and delivery with the agenda built 'out of the subjective, embodied experience of illness or caring for someone who is ill' (2003, 20). Just as efforts are needed, and made, to find the point of balance organisationally and institutionally, the boundary lines in the relationship between lay and palliative care communities need to be drawn in order to find the point of balance.

Foucault (1976) has made explicit the dynamic of power that may exist in relationships, and in the development of his observations on pastoral power (1982) has highlighted the potential for even deeper, but more subtle, probing of the individual. The positive perception of palliative care services, in contrast to general health care services, suggests that individuals like a more personal approach but begs a question as to whether this can be too personal at times. The comments made by some patients to the nursing staff reflect a resistance to questioning. The reluctance of some families to avail of palliative care services until the last minute may also be a form of resistance.

An appropriate level of involvement between patients, family members and staff is somewhere along a continuum of privacy and intrusion, a balance understood by one of the home care nurses as she described that it was okay to think about patients at ten in the evening but not okay to ring to check they were okay. Likewise, the midway point between acceptance and denial of impending death is about 'helping people accept the fact that they are dying and not "acceptance" as in being happy about it', as one of the doctors in this study identified. In a culture of Catholicism, where religious and spiritual discourses are prominent within many social activities, a question must be raised as to whether there is a line between 'accompaniment' and 'being led' and a point of balance needs to be identified.

Elias (1985) has stated that dying is a largely unformed blank area on the social map. In drawing these fine lines and the intersections between communities, some of these blank areas may begin to be sketched.

Revisiting cartography

A conceptual framework of cartography has been used as a backdrop throughout this research. Harley (1988) has likened cartography to a 'form of knowledge and form of power', and using a cartographic framework in this research has enabled the dynamics of the social relationships to become more explicit. Using an analogy of landscape and the relationships of topographical features also serves to make the relationship with and between the social actors within their communities more visible.

Social maps

A 'good death' has been considered as simultaneously an individual and a social experience. Within the individual experience of death and dying there is also a uniquely individual aspect and a social aspect. The point at which the individual meets with family members, professional staff and the organisation is the point of intersection where death, good or otherwise, becomes a social experience. Following on from the earlier discussions, this intersection has the potential to form a supportive arch, as intersecting lines do in finding their angle of repose.

The angle of repose

The angle of repose is a term within physics to describe 'the inclination of a plane at which a body placed on the plane would remain at rest, or if in motion would roll or slide down with uniform velocity; the angle at which the various kinds of earth will stand when abandoned to themselves'. *The New Oxford Dictionary of English* (1998 edition) offers this meaning: 'the steepest angle at which a sloping surface formed of loose material is stable'.

Wallace Stegnar, in a novel entitled *Angle of repose* (1992, first published in 1971), relates a story of discovery—personal, historical and geographical—in which the story of the lives of the narrator's grandparents is rediscovered and told. At the end of the novel, the narrator explains his use of the term 'angle of repose' in relation to his grandmother's life. He explains that 'it was the angle at which a man or a woman finally lies down' (1992, 568) and continues that he had hoped to find, in his exploration of the lives of his grandparents,

> *'another angle in all those years when she was growing old and older and very old, and my Grandfather was matching her year for year. A separate line that did not intersect with hers. They were vertical people, they lived by pride and it is only by the ocular illusion of perspective that they can be said to have met. But he had not been dead two months when she lay down and died too, and that may indicate that at that absolute vanishing point they did intersect.... some hopeful cowardly geometer in my brain tells me that it [the angle of repose] is the angle at which two lines prop each other up, the leaning-together from the vertical which produces the false arch. For lack of a keystone, the false arch may*

> *be as much as one can expect in this life. Only the very lucky discover the keystone.'*

So it is in this sense that the angle of repose is used in these social maps—the intersection of the lives of individuals and the way they support each other. Sometimes this placing together produces the false or temporary arch that Stegnar talks of, sufficient unto its purpose; the lucky, as Stegnar says, find in this false arch a keystone. In drawing these social maps the configuration of lines, or lives, can produce these arches, not only between people but also between larger social groups.

A social landscape

The social landscape is occupied by social actors, just as topographical features occupy the physical landscape. This social landscape may be fragile or robust, just like the physical landscape.

The relationship between the landscape and modern technology needs to be handled with care and can, if handled sensitively, be a positive intervention. Likewise, in the social landscape, the interventions of the professional staff in caring for the dying person and family members can also be positive interventions. It is in this context that Clark's (1999) assertion that 'total pain' is something of an imperialistic notion has particular relevance. While the concept of 'total pain' potentially humanises physical suffering and in freeing patients from physical pain can provide access to their other problems, mental, spiritual and social, it also has the potential to be overly invasive, as Clark argues. The dynamics of relationships that have been previously suggested lend themselves to considering this concept in these terms. The positions of visitors and occupiers are particularly relevant in terms of a social landscape. The concept of total pain, sensitively and appropriately applied, does have the potential to ease suffering. On the other hand, if applied over-rigorously, it has—like the surveying tools that probe even the soul, as Clark describes—the potential to probe too deeply, changing the dynamic within these social relationships from visitor and occupier to coloniser and colonised, with all the ensuing problems (Nandy 1983).

The positions of visitors and occupiers are interchangeable, depending on whose home is being visited, and this has been a useful way to consider the relationships between patients, families and professional staff. Being a visitor, however, has responsibilities. There are social manners to be observed, which, when transgressed, can be problematic. The lines between surveillance and observation, privacy and intrusion, accompaniment and being led, person-focused care or being too personal, made visible earlier in this discussion, are very fine and need to be walked with poise and balance, as they are drawn differently by each patient and each family.

Fractals on the social landscape—the uniquely individual experience of dying

There is a part of the experience of death and dying that is uniquely individual. The cartographer Tim Robinson has written on the mapping of south Connemara in the west of Ireland, an area that features a particularly rugged coastline (Robinson 1996). Robinson's method of map-making involves an intimacy with the physical landscape, and he describes his map of Connemara as 'a record of a long walk, an intimate, knotted, itinerary that visits each place within its territory' (1996, 81). In attempting to record and measure the rugged coastline of south Connemara, he became aware of the work of an American mathematician, Benoit Mandelbrot, who has proved that an outline as complex as a coastline does not have a definable length. The idea that better approximation of its length is possible by finer and finer detail is false; the series of approximations 'does not converge to an answer, it just gets bigger and bigger, to infinity' (*op. cit.*, 81).

The coastline that Robinson attempted to measure is composed of forms that Mandelbrot has called fractals, derived from the Latin *fractus*, meaning broken. It is based on the idea of non-integral dimensionality—i.e. a geometric form that has more than one dimension and less than two. Mandelbrot combined the notion of non-integrated dimensionality with the fact that coastlines are virtually infinitely long to create the idea of fractals, which is a unit of measurement that is infinite.

Robinson, whose background as a mathematician has given him an ease with which to talk about these concepts, states that although it may appear absurd to consider dimensionality in terms of 1.5 or 2.7, in fact these concepts are a feature of many natural features from curdled milk to coastlines, systems of geological faults, cloud forms and even the distribution of the 200 billion galaxies in space (*op. cit.*, 83).

Robinson has described the coastline of south Connemara as composed of fractals that are infinite and therefore ultimately unmappable, although the generality of the landscape can be mapped. In much the same way, the uniquely individual aspect of the experience of death and dying is ultimately unknowable, although, like the Connemara coastline that Robinson discusses, the generality of the experience can be understood. In this way, the person who is dying can be considered, in terms of a social map, as akin to this part of the coastline, a fractal in the social landscape. While the fractals in the coastline may be unmappable, except in a general sense, they are related to and part of the physical landscape. So too is the individual.

The hinterland

Just as the unique aspect of the individual can be represented as a fractal on the coastline, this is part of a greater landscape, a hinterland. The communities identified earlier can be located on this social map—firstly the community within which the individual resides, which in turn intersects with, for the purpose of this discussion, the palliative care community. As discussed earlier, the palliative care community intersects with others, such as the health service, and some palliative communities, although not all, also intersect with Catholic religious orders. These intersections can be drawn on and on, building up a social map that charts the social institutions and their relationship with each other and the way in which they intersect with the lives of individuals and their social worlds. Social maps of this kind may have a wider application, and thus different communities in different alignments may intersect each other.

Robinson has also discovered in his exploration of fractals 'that the general characteristics are the same, roughly speaking, at all scales, from the whole side of

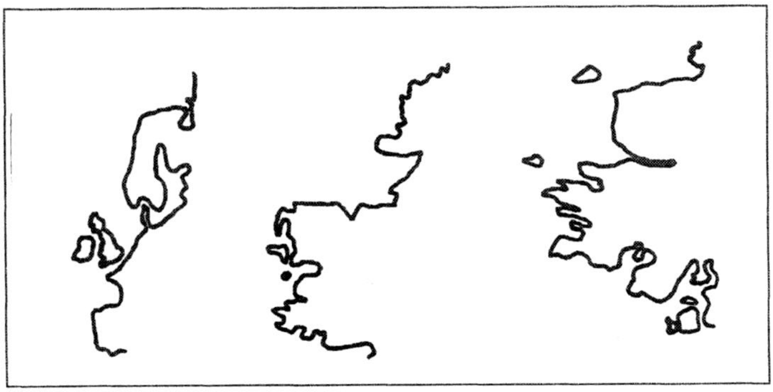

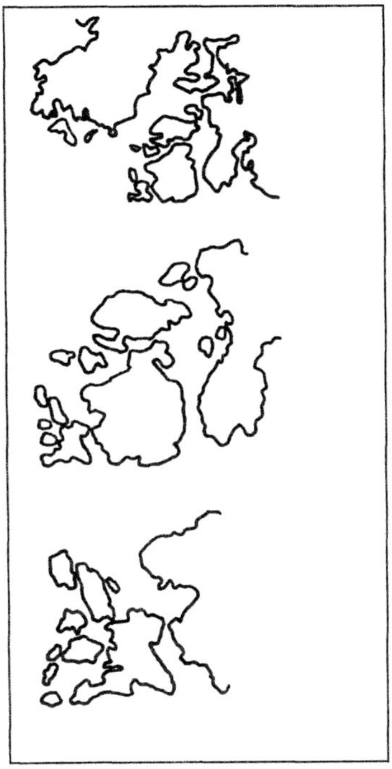

Above—Self-similiar shapes.

Left—Fractals, on the coastline of south Connemara.

Illustrations from 'A Connemara fractal' in Robinson 1996.

a continent down to the margins of a rock pool' (1996, 82). These shapes are described as 'self-similar'. Using the analogy of fractals again and the idea of self-similar shapes, the dimensions of the social communities can also be considered as self-similar, although, like the coastline, not duplications. For instance, communities and societies are comprised of individuals who when grouped together as communities form a 'self-similar' shape of multiple individuals (or fractals). The illustration (on the previous page, from Robinson 1996) shows how the coastline of western Europe mirrors, but is not a duplication of, the coastline of south Connemara. Similarly, the illustration of fractals on the Connemara coast suggests how these fractals or individuals may be viewed as distinct yet integrated into the surrounding landscape or social groups.

As yet, the social maps drawn here are sketchy attempts to fill the blank area that Elias has observed. The discussion of the wider community that may form part of the social world of the terminally ill patient has suggested that the presence of deceased relatives and friends may form part of their social world. Barbato *et al.* (1999) have argued that, however experiences such as deathbed visions and a 'sense of presence' may be understood, they are real for the person who has them. On a social map they could be considered as a dotted line, a tentative sketch of a further potential social world. The numerous accounts of near-death experiences in which people supposedly return from death with a changed world-view, having, as Kellehear (2000a) has observed, perceived a form of 'utopian society', offer a tantalising hint that there may be other social worlds currently unmappable.

Revisiting ethics

The ethical considerations involved in social research, in particular the ethical considerations for conducting research in palliative care and more specifically the issue of interviewing terminally ill patients, were discussed in Chapter 3. The original proposal and agreement for the research included interviews with terminally ill patients. The attempts to interview patients for this research were also outlined, and I stated that, as the research progressed, I began to have a growing sense of unease about whether interviewing patients was actually appropriate.

The arguments presented by de Raeve (1994) raise pertinent questions, especially concerning the irreconcilable perspectives of the researcher and the subject. In writing the research proposals I used the compelling arguments for interviewing patients that have appeared in the published literature (Hinton 1980; McDonnell 1989; Cartwright and Seale 1990; Higginson *et al.* 1990; Kellehear 1990; Dand *et al.* 1991; Field *et al.* 1993; Spillar and Alexander 1993; Townsend 1993; Field 1995). I mentioned de Raeve in the initial proposal as a counter-argument but in reality I paid little heed to her view. As the research progressed, however, I found myself returning again and again to the issues that she and others, such as Kellehear (1989; 1998), have raised in relation to the inclusion of terminally ill people in research.

From the outset of the research I was aware that palliative care is a sensitive area for social research and, as outlined in the methodology, the provision of support for participants was addressed prior to and during the research. I had adopted a strategy of leaving the interviews with patients until later in the research as I wanted to establish trustworthiness. This strategy worked as I was given permission to interview anyone in the hospice, including patients in the in-patient unit.

As the research progressed and I spent more time in the hospice, I became reluctant to pursue patient interviews although there was considerable pressure to do so. This pressure was internal, i.e. from me in pursuit of the research goals, a real pressure that forms part of de Raeve's argument on irreconcilable perspectives. There was also pressure from some members of staff who were highly committed to the research and as a result anxious for me to meet the research goals. Because of my reluctance I was asked, by a senior member of staff, whether I was uncomfortable about conducting interviews with people who were dying, and although it was not stated I sensed that this was a question about whether I was 'up to it'. The truth was that I was uncomfortable—not because I was afraid to interview dying people but because of a growing unease about the appropriateness of doing so, although it took a number of months for me to understand why I felt it was inappropriate.

Conflicting perspectives

De Raeve discusses the difficulties inherent in the research process of subjects becoming a means to an end, which are essentially the researcher's ends, not the subjects'. She considers that in qualitative research methodologies researchers may not perceive themselves to be treating subjects in this way; this type of research often uses terms such as 'collaborator' or 'informant' for their subjects, and researchers can consider themselves as having a partnership with the people studied (1994, 300). But as de Raeve argues, if this was truly the case it would mean that the research subject 'co-authored the report and that both parties had a right of veto about what was to be said and whether or not publication should take place and if so where' (*op. cit.*, 300). She acknowledges that safeguards and sensitive interviewing are important in qualitative research methodologies but argues that these do little to alter the fundamental positions of researcher and subject.

Informed consent is one safeguard used to counteract the 'means–end treatment of research subjects', particularly, as de Raeve argues, when the research subject can identify with the researcher's goals rather than be simply compliant. Nevertheless, de Raeve also queried whether patients who are already experiencing vulnerability and dependency in a health care setting are not already compromised to some degree in relation to health care professionals (*op. cit.*, 301)—and, I would add, social researchers.

Following on from this argument concerning the opposing perspectives of researcher and subject, de Raeve specifically considers the issue of interviewing terminally ill people. Within palliative care, de Raeve argues, supporting and caring for patients appears to be antithetical to the research idea that one is enlisting patients to support the researcher's goals. This juxtaposition of positions, she argues, is heightened if one considers that 'in the process of dying, people may be slowly disengaging from the world, whereas a research enquiry seems to require the opposite: that people remain engaged and do not slip away' (op. cit., 302).

Some studies give credence to de Raeve's view, as patients admitted to a hospice in-patient unit will generally be at an advanced stage of their illness. Cohen *et al.* (2001) have noted in a study of quality-of-life changes following admission to palliative care units that of 1131 patients admitted 51% were not well enough to complete the initial questionnaire on admission; 135 people completed the first McGill Quality of Life Questionnaire (MQOL). Of the total number of admissions, only 32 patients had 'sufficient energy' to complete all stages of the research, which included a second questionnaire a week after admission and a subsequent semi-structured interview.

A study of suffering and comfort at the end of life (Olsen *et al.* 2001) also supports de Raeve's view of the patient disengaging from the world. Morse (2002), reporting on this study, describes a state of 'endurance' experienced by patients, which, she argues, enables patients to prioritise, conserve energy, remain focused and thus 'bear the unbearable'. Olsen *et al.* (2001) have described this state as 'cocooning', in which the individuals' focus becomes increasingly internalised and they restrict contact with others, expending energy on family and closest friends: 'their world slowly becomes encapsulated, reduced to only those parts that are essential'. A traditional view of the final 48 hours of life is still influential in Spain, according to Fainsinger *et al.* (2003), who state that the last 48 hours of life for a dying patient are still the time of the *agonía*. The *agonía* has been defined, since the fifteenth century, as 'the space of time that takes place between the clouding of the sense and the departure of the soul' (*ibid.*, 47).

There are considerable counter-arguments that can be presented against de Raeve's position and she certainly elicited a vociferous response from Balfour Mount and others (Mount *et al.* 1995) who took issue with many of the points she raised, including her distinction between the living and the dying, as already discussed in Chapter 3. Mount *et al.* argue that de Raeve's suggestion that terminally ill patients be disqualified as research participants owing to frailty is demeaning and unacceptable. Others, such as Kellehear (1989), argue that there is certainly a case that without information and without questioning there is only speculation and opinion, and without information about what may be typical or normal people may feel that their own experiences are unusual or deviant (Kellehear 1989, 65). But

Kellehear (1998, 16) also argued that research is always about interfering with people and that some way of minimising that interference needs to be found.

My own experience of attempting to include patients in the research highlighted the issues that de Raeve has raised. One patient was interviewed for this study, although two others were approached for inclusion. It is not possible to make any general statements about patients' experience based on one interview and two preliminary conversations, but the interview and conversations in themselves suggest that while patients may want 'someone to talk to' (Jarrett *et al.* 1999), what they may wish to talk about may not be directly related to the research. The preliminary conversations that I had with patients to explain the research—one patient was in day care and the other was in the in-patient unit—were pleasant interactions as well as being focused on information-giving on my part. On returning to both these patients after a week, the patient in day care initially agreed to take part but any attempts at steering the conversation toward the research topic met with resistance and a return to 'everyday' conversation, much of which included his pleasure at coming to the day centre for 'the dinner' and the company. The patient in the in-patient unit was firmly against taking part in the research. I subsequently discovered, by piecing together disparate pieces of information from interviews with nursing staff, that this patient, who had been in the in-patient unit for a considerable time, had 'done all the talking he was going to do'. The patient that I did speak with, although he happily agreed to take part, also displayed a resistance to talking on the research topic and constantly returned to 'everyday' topics. As the interview progressed, I gave up trying to steer the talk in the direction of the research and we subsequently enjoyed a chat about horse racing, something which was a great source of pleasure to him and of interest to me.

On reflection, these interactions with patients probably said more about the perspective of the patients than any conversation about 'a good death' or 'comfort' or 'religion' or whatever. We talked about what was important and of interest to them, and these were not things that were 'important' to me—like spirituality or spiritual care. At the time I thought that these interactions did not meet my research goals; with hindsight it is easier to see that they did—it was simply a more circuitous and ultimately more enlightening route.

De Raeve talks about dying people disengaging from the world and how this is in conflict with the researchers' goals. This potential juxtaposition of perspectives became very real for me as I spent more and more time at the hospice. The reality of vulnerable patients and family, and indeed staff, on an everyday basis is very different to a theoretical understanding of sensitive research in palliative care and was tangible from my observations and interviews. No matter how familiar I became with the hospice and the in-patient unit, I was still taken aback every time I walked down the corridor and, through doors left slightly ajar, caught glimpses of patients near death. One participant talked about the whole 'beyondedness' of death and dying, which was a made-up phrase that could have jarred but somehow did not, and it seemed to capture some sense of what I was perceiving.

Whilst conducting the research I was reading *Hunting Mister Heartbreak*, an account by travel writer and novelist Jonathan Raban, who followed the route of European emigrants to North America by re-enacting a voyage on a cargo ship from Liverpool to New York (Raban 1990). Raban explores, in what is described as a 'map of change', his perception of changes—physical, emotional and philosophical—along the journey. Two days away from land he writes:

> '*It must have been at just this point of the voyage that the migrants, lately emigrants, found themselves slipping into their new characters as immigrants—comers-to, not goers-away from. From here on in, you could begin to sketch your new life to yourself, to fill the obscure vacancy of "America" with solid objects. Somewhere west of Flemish Cap in the North Atlantic Basin, Paradise, Kansas acquired a barn, a fence, a herd of cows with shitty tails, a loghouse, a spread table*' (1990, 40).

The idea of people who were dying as comers-to rather than goers-away from stuck, and while there is no reason not to talk to comers-to it seemed to me that terminally ill patients and myself as researcher were occupying very different and possibly irreconcilable places. This idea of emigrants and immigrants is also a way to consider the individuality of the experience of dying and fits with the concept of the uniquely individual aspects of death as a fractal of the coastline, just described. Raban felt this change from emigrant to immigrant about two days from landfall; other emigrants may have felt this sooner and looked forward to 'Paradise, Kansas' from early on in the voyage, just as Sally's aunt looked forward to meeting her twin and other sisters again after her death, while other emigrants may never have been transformed into immigrants, except in the sense of a technical change in status.

Appropriate questions

De Raeve also queries what kind of questions we can ask of dying people, and this was part of my difficulty which the initial permission to talk to patients in day care highlights. It is now clear that day care involves a delicate balancing of frequently conflicting aims, as discussed earlier. The Field and Copp (1999) study clearly shows a shift toward conditional awareness, as discussed in Chapter 1, and day care possibly facilitates that level of awareness, allowing a minimal contact with the hospice and the full reality of impending death while at the same time helping people to stay at home as long as possible.

Patients at different stages of the dying trajectory may be unable to answer the kind of questions being asked; for instance, day care patients may be entirely focused on 'living with cancer' rather than the experience of dying. The questions that I wished to address to patients concerned a 'good death', an issue that many patients might not yet have even considered or have a wish to consider. Although participation in the research was, of course, voluntary, it seemed to me that including patients inappropriately in the research in pursuit of my research goals was not ethical research.

De Raeve also comments that although we do not tend to phrase research questions along such lines as 'What is it like to be dying?' this may nevertheless be part of our implicit agenda (1994, 302). At the back of my mind, no matter how skilfully I phrased questions about the needs people may have and whether religion and family were a comfort and so on, I could not escape a feeling that what I was really asking was 'Now you are dying, what is that like?'

A cultural difference

Field (1995) has argued that enough studies have been conducted which have included terminally ill patients to discount a view that these patients should not be interviewed. Again, while writing the research proposal this was the argument I used, and again as the research progressed I began to query this. Another way of considering this is to ask 'If enough studies have been done, why do more?' The social isolation of dying patients and the need to gain understanding of the needs of dying people which prompted much of the early research with terminally ill patients may have changed with the addition of palliative care services, both in hospices and in other health care services.

Much of the palliative care research with terminally ill patients has been undertaken in the UK, and little or no research has been undertaken with terminally ill patients in Ireland. While this may appear a compelling reason for doing such research, considerable cultural differences exist. As I spent time in the hospice I became increasingly aware of the difference between what I was observing and what was documented in the literature, a literature that is based mainly on palliative care experiences in the UK and elsewhere and which has been described in earlier chapters.

What I was observing in the hospice was not, as the ethical justifications portray, isolated patients who needed someone to hear their story and listen to their needs. Instead, I observed dying patients surrounded by many family members, who often undertook long vigils at the bedside, and professional staff, whose attention on the patient and the family members was extremely concentrated. The social world of the dying person in the hospice sometimes seemed a very crowded place, prompting me to question whether there was room for a researcher and whether there were already enough people listening.

A microcosm of the research

With hindsight it is much easier to see that the unease I was feeling about including terminally ill people in the research had to do with the core themes of the research—the differences between perspectives, the nature of relationships, identifying boundaries and the lines that demarcate them, and the distinction between the uniquely individual aspects of a 'good death' and the social aspects of a 'good death'. In a sense, the difficulty that I had with interviewing patients and the issues I have addressed here are a microcosm of the whole research.

De Raeve has made explicit the relationship between researcher and subject. The discussion on relationships, earlier in this chapter, considers the dynamics involved, the terms of negotiation and the delicate line between potentially opposing views. These issues are also present between the researcher and participants. Although subjects and researchers have different perspectives, the lay and professional perspectives highlighted in this research have shown that a difference in perspective does not mean they are necessarily mutually exclusive. The way in which professionals care for patients is not necessarily at variance with the needs of patients and family members, although the professional practice of palliative care may not always exactly fit with patients and family members and some degree of negotiation and accommodation is present from both perspectives.

In revisiting ethical considerations concerning interviewing terminally ill patients I am not suggesting that interviewing patients *per se* is unethical; clearly there is a real need to understand the perspectives of patients and family members. In Ireland, the historical development of the health service, discussed previously, has been a dominant discourse from powerful lobbies and not from patients and their families; similarly, in the emergence of a more individualistic society in Ireland there is a need to hear more individual voices. The social map just described clearly has large blank areas.

Nevertheless, I am saying that this is more complex than it may at first appear. Ethical principles are a guideline, not permission slips, and ethical decision-making is an ongoing part of conducting research. This ongoing process is the same as the process involved in the relationships between health care professionals, patients and family members, as already discussed. Distinguishing and making explicit the uniquely individual and the social aspects of death and dying clarifies to some extent who can be included in research, what questions can be asked, and when it is appropriate to ask them.

De Raeve comments that it is likely that we are all curious about death and the process of dying, and the less this can be answered the more curious we may become. She argues, however, that there may be questions that are always fundamentally unanswerable, and some questions about death and the process of dying may be among them; she states that perhaps the only respectful position is to 'simply and gratefully receive what is generously and spontaneously offered' (*op. cit.*, 302). This is reminiscent of La Rochefoucald's famous observation that it is impossible to look directly at the sun or at death (cited in Small 1997, 210). There are aspects and characteristics of death and dying that we can understand in much the same way that we can understand and have information about the sun, but the experience of the sun on the skin is each person's own experience. Perhaps an understanding of death and dying can only be given and not looked for directly; perhaps death always and ultimately remains a mystery and a secret (Derrida 1995).

Summary

This chapter has considered the relationships that are at the heart of palliative care. Kellehear (2002) has identified the dying person as residing within a social community, a community that provides support and is the location for many of the tasks that need to be accomplished before death. This study has extended the view of community and identified that professionals also reside within their own communities, which have specific cultural values and beliefs.

The role of patients, relatives and professional staff as visitors and occupiers in different locations makes explicit the dynamics of power that exist within these relationships. Palliative care is person-focused but this focus also has the potential to be too focused. The manners of engagement within this person-focused relationship demand that the boundary lines between aspects such as privacy and intrusion need to be clearly identified. The angle of repose—the point at which the lines of intersection support one another—needs to be sought within these relationships.

Elias identified a blank area of the social map of death and dying and this study has attempted to fill in some of these blank areas. A 'good death' was considered as simultaneously a uniquely individual experience and a social experience. An analogy has been drawn between the infinitely immeasurable and ultimately unknowable fractals on the coastal landscape and points of intersection between that coastline and the surrounding landscape. Viewed in this way, the individual retains his or her unique aspects while at the same time can be understood as being located in, and as part of, a wider social world.

A return was made to the ethical decision-making that formed a part of this research. The decision not to include patients as part of the research was re-examined in the light of ethical arguments about the appropriateness of including terminally ill patients in research. The potentially opposing positions of patients and researchers were, in hindsight, seen to reflect the emerging themes of the study. Just as the fine lines that demarcate boundaries between health care professionals and patients and relatives need to be made explicit and a point of balance needs to be found, a point of balance between the researcher, the aims of the research, the potential positive outcome of research and the perspective of the participants also needs to be made explicit and be clearly identified.

CHAPTER 11
Conclusion

This book set out to explore understandings of a 'good death' and the spiritual dimension of care in an Irish palliative care setting and to explore the cultural, social and policy contexts that shape understandings. Exploration, cartography and map-making formed the conceptual framework and while this began as a useful organising principle it became a central focus and ultimately provided greater understanding and clarity for filling in the blank areas on the social map that Elias (1985, 28) identified. This social map has identified points of intersection between social actors and social institutions in the context of care for the dying in Ireland.

Elias (*op. cit*) has suggested that it is our task to 'make the end, the parting from human beings, when it comes, as easy and as pleasant as possible, for others as well as ourselves'. A 'good death' is about the 'manner of parting' and the tasks that need to be accomplished in order to make that as easy and as pleasant as possible. It was clear from the historical and contemporary representations of a 'good death' that how these tasks are defined and accomplished changes over time and across cultures.

I have considered 'the manner of parting' within Irish palliative care, where traditional beliefs and practices around death and dying in Ireland continue to be important although some are now changing. Some commentators have argued that in Ireland a different cosmology exists, one that views another and powerful realm in close connection with this world. While this may be the case, the predominant position of the Catholic Church in Ireland, and its central role in social institutions since the nineteenth century, suggests that the way in which beliefs or understandings of this cosmology are expressed is mainly through a cultural lens shaped by Catholicism. The influence of the Catholic Church is now considerably diminished and recent research suggests that there is a parallel and secular discourse emerging and that Ireland is characterised by a 'changing landscape' (Keegan and van Doorslaer 2001).

The preliminary research focus—exploring nearing death awareness (NDA)—was altered as I felt that there were more fundamental questions to be explored. This change of direction, toward an understanding of a 'good death' and spiritual care within a palliative care setting, incorporated some aspects of NDA, such as visions of deceased relatives, but experiences can best be understood within the context of relationship.

Relationships with and between individuals, professional staff and health care organisations are influenced and shaped by the social and historical context within which they are situated. In Ireland, these relationships reflect the legacy of the past. There is a positive perception of the person-focused approach of palliative care, although this positive perception must be considered in the context of an inequitable and under-resourced health service. If, as I have argued, relationship is at the heart of palliative care, there is a need to make explicit the nature of this relationship and to make explicit the power relationships that exist.

A 'good death' is simultaneously an individual and a social experience. As a social experience, there are multiple needs that require consideration—those of the dying person, relatives, professional staff and the organisation. The social world of the dying person, consisting of multiple social actors and institutions, can be a crowded place. In palliative care, the multi-disciplinary team working of the model that serves to provide holistic care also adds to the webs of interaction.

Kellehear (2002) has drawn attention to the social community within which the dying person is situated. Throughout life people are part of their own social community—of friends and relatives—and it is within this social community that many of the tasks for the parting to be 'as easy and pleasant' as possible need to take place. I have extended Kellehear's idea of community to include those of the professional and other staff, such as the palliative care service and other institutions such as the health service. In considering all these groups as separate communities, rather than as lay and professional perspectives, it becomes clearer that each community has its own beliefs and values, its own culture, which may sometimes fit with others but can also conflict.

The adoption of cartography as a means for exploring the understandings of a 'good death' and spiritual care has, as Lefebvre (1991) suggested, provided a unity between disparate levels and has shown more clearly where these merge, connect or even collide, to borrow Lefebvre's phrase. Examining relationships according to the location of care has shown more clearly where there are connections and where there are possible points of collision. Understanding the relationships in terms of visitors and occupiers also makes more explicit the dynamics of these relationships and the manners of engagement.

The 'community' of palliative care stands in close relationship to the social community of the dying person because of the person-focused approach of the model. This, however, does not mean that these communities have identical or even similar cultural beliefs or values, although this may sometimes be the case. The holistic view of patients that is a hallmark of palliative care is a welcome initiative in health care but it brings additional responsibilities. There is a need to understand that while palliative care is person-focused, it is health care and as such it is a professional health care community with specific objectives.

Small (2003, 20) has argued for the reconciliation of institutional and professional agendas and the subjective embodied experience of illness or caring for someone who is ill; part of this reconciliation is understanding the boundary lines between the different communities. While hospices strive to be home-like they are not the patient's home, and while the professional and other staff adopt a friendly approach they are not the patient's personal friends. In adopting a holistic approach to patients and family members these boundaries can sometimes become blurred and are difficult for members of each of the communities to identify clearly. Care is needed to ensure that the person-focused approach does not become too personal and that the very fine lines, for instance between privacy and intrusion and between accompaniment and being led, are understood.

I have attempted to fill in some of the blank areas of the social map of death and dying that Elias identified. The uniquely individual aspect of the experience of dying has been considered as akin to the fragmented coastal landscape—as a fractal on this landscape. While the uniquely individual aspect is always ultimately unknowable, individuals (and coastlines) are part of a larger landscape and communities are located within this hinterland. The intersections between the individual and their community can be identified, and in turn the intersections between this social community and other social institutions can also be identified.

Descriptions of lay ideas of health and illness as a 'warp and weft' (Seymour 1999) and 'as historical strata laid down by a culture in motion' (Williamson 1990) point to the potential of drawing social maps that are highly textured, complex and multi-dimensional. At present the social map identified in this study is no more than a rough sketch.

BIBLIOGRAPHY

Abu-Saad, H. (2001) *Evidence-based palliative care: across the life span*. Oxford. Blackwell Science.

Addington-Hall, J. and Higginson, A. (eds) (2001) *Palliative care for non-cancer patients*. Oxford University Press.

—— and McCarthy, M. (1995) 'Regional study of care for the dying: methods and sample characteristics', *Palliative Medicine* **9**, 27–35.

Ainsworth-Smith, I. (1998) 'The spiritual and pastoral dimension of chaplaincy work', *Journal of Interpersonal Care* **12** (4), 380–7.

Albery, N., Elliot, G. and Elliot, J. (eds) (1993) *The Natural Death Handbook*. London. Virgin.

Albinsson, L. and Strang, P. (2003) 'Differences in supporting families of dementia patients and cancer patients: a palliative perspective', *Palliative Medicine* **17**, 359–67.

Alderson, P. (1995) *Listening to children: children, ethics and social research*. Ilford. Barnardos.

Allen, D. (2000) 'Negotiating the role of expert carers on an adult hospital ward', *Sociology of Health and Illness* **22**, 149–71.

Ariès, P. (1994) *Western attitudes toward death from the Middle Ages to the present* (pbk edn). London. Marion Boyars Publishers.

Arksey, H. and Knight, P. (1999) *Interviewing for social scientists*. London. Sage Publications.

Arney, W. and Bergen, B. (1984) *Medicine and the management of living: taming the last great beast*. University of Chicago Press.

Aston, M. (1994) 'Death', in R. Horrox (ed.), *Fifteenth-century attitudes: perceptions of life in late medieval England* 35–52. Cambridge University Press.

Babler, J. E. (1997) 'A comparison of spiritual care provided by Hospice social workers, nurses and spiritual care professionals', *The Hospice Journal* **12** (4). Haworth Press.

Baines, M. (1990) 'Tackling Total Pain', in C. Saunders (ed.), *Hospice and palliative care: an interdisciplinary approach*, 123–42. London. Edward Arnold.

Baird, R. M. (1985) 'Meaning in life: discovered or created?', *Journal of Religion and Health* **24**, 2.

Barbato, M., Blunden, C., Reid, N., Irwin, H. and Rodriques, P. (1999) 'Parapsychological phenomena near the time of death', *Journal of Palliative Care* **15** (2), 30–7.

Barrett, W. (1926) *Death-bed visions*. London. Methuen.

Barrington, R. (1987) *Health, medicine and politics 1900–1970*. Dublin. Institute of Public Administration.

Barthes, R. (1993) *Mythologies*. London. Vintage.

Bartley, C. (2001) 'Ars Moriendi', in G. Howarth and O. Leaman, *Encyclopedia of death and dying*, 31. London. Routledge.

Basford, T. (1990) *Near-death experiences: an annotated bibliography*. New York and London. Garland Publishing.

Batchelor, J. and Briggs, C. (1994) 'Subject, project or self? Thoughts on ethical dilemmas for social and medical research', *Social Science and Medicine* **39** (7), 949–54.

Beauchamp, T., Faden, R., Wallace, R. J. and Walters, L. (1982) 'Introduction', in T. Beauchamp, R. Faden and R. Wallace (eds), *Ethical issues in social science research* 10–14. Baltimore. John Hopkins University Press.

Bennett, G. (1987) *Traditions of belief: women, folklore and the supernatural today*. London. Penguin.

Berger, P. (1997) 'Epistemological modesty', *Christian Century* **114**, 972–5.

Biswas, B. (1993) 'A nurse's view', in D. Clark (ed.), *The future for palliative care*, 142–67. Buckingham. Open University Press.

Blaxter, M. (1990) *Health and lifestyles*. London. Routledge.

—— and Paterson, E. (1982) *Mothers and daughter: a three-generational study of health attributes and behaviour*. London. Heinemann.

Bloch, M. and Parry, J. (1982) *Death and the regeneration of life*. Cambridge

University Press.

Blunt, A. and Rose, G. (1994) 'Introduction: women's colonial and post colonial geographies', in A. Blunt and G. Rose (eds), *Writing women and space* 5–16. New York and London. The Guildford Press.

Bolster, E. (1979) *The Knights of Columbanus*. Dublin. Gill and Macmillan.

Boud, D., Keogh, R. and Walker, D. (1985) 'Promoting reflection in learning: a model', in D. Boud, R. Keogh and D. Walker (eds), *Reflection: turning experience into learning*, 18–35. London. Kogan Page.

Bowling, A. (1997) *Research methods in health: investigating health and health services*. Buckingham. Open University Press.

Bown, J. and Williams, A. (1993) 'Spirituality and nursing: a review of the literature', *Journal of Advances in Health and Nursing Care* **2** (4), 41–66.

Bradbury, M. (1999) *Representations of death: a social psychological perspective*. London. Routledge.

Bradshaw, A. (1996a) 'Lighting the lamp: the covenant as an encompassing framework for the spiritual dimension of nursing care', in E. S. Farmer (ed.), *Exploring the spiritual dimension in caring*, 27–39. Salisbury. Quay.

—— (1996b) 'The spiritual dimension of hospice: the secularisation of an ideal', *Social Science and Medicine* **43** (3), 409–19.

Breen, M. (2001) 'The forest is on fire', in M. Breen (ed.), *A fire in the forest: religious life in Ireland* 26–43. Dublin. Veritas Publications.

Breen, R., Hannan, D., Rottman, D. and Whelan, C. (1990) *Understanding contemporary Ireland: state, class and development in the Republic of Ireland*. London. Macmillan.

Brewis, K. (2003) 'A matter of life and death', *Sunday Times Magazine*, 10 August, 42–7.

Browne, N. (1986) *Against the tide*. Dublin. Gill and Macmillan.

Burgess, R. (1985) 'The whole truth? Some ethical problems of research in a comprehensive school', in R. G. Burgess (ed.), *Strategies of educational research: qualitative methods*, 143–76. Lewes. Falmer Press.

Burnard, P. (1987) 'Spiritual distress and the nursing response: theoretical considerations and counselling skills', *Journal of Advanced Nursing* **12**, 377–82.

Butler, K. (1980) *We help them home: a history of Our Lady's Hospice, Harold's Cross*. Dublin. Caritas Press.

Byrne, F. J. (1967) 'Early Irish society', in F. X. Martin and T. W. Moody (eds), *The course of Irish history*, 43–60. Cork. Mercier Press.

Callanan, M. and Keeley, P. (1997) *Final gifts: understanding the special awareness, needs and communications of the dying*. New York. Bantam Publishing.

Carr, W. (2001) 'Spirituality and religion: chaplaincy in context', in H. Orchard (ed.), *Spirituality in health care contexts,* 78–102. London. Jessica Kingsley Publishers.

Cartwright, A. and Seale, C. (1990) *The natural history of a survey: an account of the methodological issues encountered in a study of life before death*. London. King Edward's Hospital Fund for London.

Central Statistics Office (2007) *Equality in Ireland 2007*. Dublin. Stationery Office.

Charmaz, K. (1980) *The social reality of death: death in contemporary America*. Reading, Massachusetts. Addison-Wesley.

—— and Mitchell, R. (2001) 'Grounded Theory and ethnography', in P. Atkinson, A. Coffey, C. Delamont, J. Lofland and L. Lofland (eds), *Handbook of ethnography* 197–213, London. Sage Publications.

Clark, D. (1982) *Between pulpit and pew: folk religion in a North Yorkshire fishing village*. Cambridge University Press.

—— (1999) '"Total Pain": disciplinary power and the body in the work of Cicely Saunders, 1958–1967', *Social Science and Medicine* **49**, 727–36.

—— (2000) 'Support and supervision in palliative care research', *Palliative Medicine* **14**, 441–6.

Cobb, M. (2001) *The dying soul: spiritual care at the end of life*. Buckingham. Open University Press.

Cohen, S.R., Boston, P., Mount, B.M. and Porterfield, P. (2001) 'Changes in quality of life following admission to palliative care units', *Palliative Medicine* **15**, 363–71.

Cooney, J. (1999) *John Charles McQuaid—ruler of Catholic Ireland*. Dublin. O'Brien Press.

Copp, G. (1998) 'A review of current theories of death and dying', *Journal of Advanced Nursing* **28** (2), 382–90.

Corner, J. (1996) 'Is there a research paradigm for palliative research?', *Palliative Medicine* **10**, 201–8.

Cornette, K. (1997) 'For whenever I am weak, I am strong…', *International Journal of Palliative Nursing* **3** (1), 6–13.

Corr, C., Doka, K. and Kastenbaum, R. (1999) 'Dying and its interpreters: a review of selected literature and some comments on the state of the field', *Omega* **39** (4), 239–59.

Coyle, N. (1997) 'Interdisciplinary collaboration in hospital palliative care: chimera or goal' [editorial], *Palliative Medicine* **11**, 265–6.

Czechmeister, C. (1994) 'Metaphor in illness and nursing: a two-edged sword. A discussion of the social use of metaphor in everyday language, and the implications of nursing and nursing education', *Journal of Advanced Nursing* **19**, 1226–33.

Dand, P., Field, D., Ahmedzai, S. and Biswas, B. (1991) *Client satisfaction with care at the Leicestershire Hospice* (Occasional Paper No. 2). Sheffield. Trent Palliative Care Centre.

Davey, B. (1988) 'Ethical framework of the consultation: doctor's assumption about the patient's need to know', paper given to the International Conference on Communication in Health Care, Churchill College, Cambridge, July 1988.

Davie, G. (2000) 'Religion in modern Britain: changing sociological assumptions', *Sociology* **34**, 113–28.

Davies, D. and Dodd, J. (2003) 'Qualitative research and the question of rigour', *Qualitative Health Research* **12** (2), 279–89.

De Beauvoir, S. (1966) *A very easy death*. London. Deutsch and Weidenfeld and

Nicholson.

Dein, S. (1997) 'Does being religious help or hinder coping with chronic illness? A critical literature review', *Palliative Medicine* **11**, 291–8.

Dekkers, W., Sandman, L. and Webb, P. (2002) 'Good death or good life as a goal of palliative care', in D. Clarke (ed.), *The ethics of palliative care,* 56–74. Buckingham. Open University Press.

Denzin, N. (1970) *The research act in sociology: a theoretical introduction to sociological methods*. London. Butterworths.

—— and Lincoln, Y. (2003) *Collecting and interpreting qualitative materials* (2nd edn). London. Sage Publications.

Department of Health (1994) *Shaping a healthier future*. Dublin. Stationery Office.

—— (2001) *Quality and fairness—a health system for you*. Dublin. Stationery Office.

—— (2002) *Acute hospital bed capacity: a national review*. Dublin. Stationery Office.

de Raeve, L. (1994) 'Ethical issues in palliative care research', *Palliative Medicine* **8**, 298–305.

Derrida, J. (1995) *The gift of death*. University of Chicago Press.

Dom, H. (1999) 'Spiritual care, need and pain—recognition and response', *European Journal of Palliative Care* **6**, 3.

Donnelly, S. (1999a) 'Traditions associated with dying in the west of Scotland', *Journal of Palliative Care* **15** (4), 64–9.

—— (1999b) 'Folklore associated with dying in the west of Ireland', *Palliative Medicine* **13**, 57–62.

Duarte Enes, S.P. (2003) 'An exploration of dignity in palliative care', *Palliative Medicine* **17**, 263–9.

DuBois, P. (1980) *The hospice way of death*. New York. Human Sciences Press.

Dunlop, R. and Hockley, J. M. (1998) *Hospital-based palliative care teams: the hospital–hospice interface* (2nd edn). Oxford University Press.

Durkheim, E. (1952) *Suicide: a study in sociology* (first published 1897). London.

Routledge and Keegan Paul.

Elias, N. (1978) *What is sociology?* London. Hutchinson

—— (1985) *The loneliness of the dying*. Oxford. Basil Blackwell.

—— (1987) *Involvement and detachment*. Oxford. Basil Blackwell.

Fainsinger, R., Nunez-Olante, J. M. and Demoissac, D. M. (2003) 'The cultural differences in perceived value of disclosure and cognition: Spain and Canada', *Journal of Palliative Care* **19** (1), 43–8.

Faulkner, A., Maguire, P. and Regnard, C. (1994) 'Breaking bad news—a flow diagram', *Palliative Medicine* **8**, 145–51.

Fernández-Shaw Toda, M. (1997) 'Ars Moriendi: images of death in Spanish art', *European Journal of Palliative Care* **4** (3), 164–8.

Fetterman, D. M. (1989) *Ethnography: step by step*. London. Sage.

Field, D. (1995) 'Terminal illness: views of patients and their lay carers', *Palliative Medicine* **9**, 45–54.

—— and Copp, G. (1999) 'Communication and awareness about dying in the 1990s', *Palliative Medicine* **13**, 459–68.

——, Dand, P., Ahmedzai, S. and Biswas, B. (1993) 'Lay carers of patients admitted to a hospice: how caring restricts their lives', *Journal of Health and Social Care* **1**, 161–8.

Finlay, L. (2002) 'Outing the researcher: the provenance, process and practice of reflexivity', *Qualitative Health Research* **12** (4), 531–45.

Finucane, R. C. (1984) *Appearances of the dead: a cultural history of ghosts*. London. Junction Books.

Firth, S. (1993) 'Approaches to death in Hindu and Sikh communities in Britain', in D. Dickenson and M. Johnson (eds), *Death, dying and bereavement*, 26–32. London. Sage.

—— (1996) 'The good death: attitudes of British Hindus', in G. Howarth and P. Jupp (eds), *Contemporary issues in the sociology of death, dying and disposal*, 96–116. London. Macmillan.

Foucault, M. (1976) *The birth of the clinic: an archaeology of medical perception*.

London. Tavistock.

—— (1982) 'Afterword: the subject and power', in H. Dreyfus and P. Rainbow (eds), *Michael Foucault: beyond structuralism and hermeneutics*, 214. University of Chicago Press.

Frankl, V. (1985) *Man's search for meaning*. New York. Washington Square Press.

Froggatt, K. (1997) 'Rites of passage and the hospice culture', *Mortality* **2** (2), 123–36.

Geertz, C. (1973) *The interpretation of cultures*. New York. Basic Books.

Gittings, C. (1999) 'Sacred and secular: 1558–1660', in P. Jupp and C. Gittings (eds), *Death in England: an illustrated history*, 147–73. Manchester University Press.

Glaser, B. and Strauss, A. (1965) *Awareness of dying*. Chicago. Aldine.

—— (1967) *The discovery of grounded theory: strategies for qualitative research*. Chicago. Aldine.

Government of Ireland (2003) *Commission on Financial Management and Control Systems in the Health Service*. Stationery Office. Dublin.

Green, M. (1995) *Celtic goddesses*. London. British Museum Press.

Hallam, E., Hockey, J. and Howarth, G. (1999) *Beyond the body: death and social identity*. London. Routledge.

Hammersley, M. (1990) 'What's wrong with ethnography? The myth of theoretical description', *Sociology* **24**, 597–615.

—— and Atkinson, P. (1983) *Ethnography: principles in practice*. London. Tavistock Publications.

Harley, J.B. (1988) 'Maps, knowledge and power', in D. Cosgrove and S. Daniels (eds), *The iconography of landscape*, 277–312. Cambridge University Press.

—— 1991 'Deconstructing the map', in T. J. Barnes and J. S. Duncan (eds), *Writing worlds: discourse, text and metaphor in the representation of landscape*, 231–47. London. Routledge.

Heaven, C. and Maguire, P. (1997) 'Disclosure of concerns by hospice patients and their identification by nurses', *Palliative Medicine* **11**, 283–90.

Herth, K. (1990) 'Fostering hope in terminally-ill people', *Journal of Advanced*

Nursing **15**, 1250–9.

Hewison, A. (1995) 'Nurses' power in interactions with patients', *Journal of Advanced Nursing* **21**, 75–82.

Higginson, I., Wade, A. and McCarthy, M. (1990) 'Palliative care; views of patients and their families', *British Medical Journal* **301**, 277–81.

Hinton, J. (1967) *Dying*. London. Penguin.

—— (1980) 'Whom do dying patients tell?', *British Medical Journal* **281**, 1328–30.

—— (1999) 'The progress of awareness and acceptance of dying assessed in cancer patients and their caring relatives', *Palliative Medicine* **13**, 19–25.

Hoad, P. (1991) 'Volunteers in the independent hospice movement', *Sociology of Health and Illness* **13** (2), 231–48.

Hockey, J. (1990) *Experiences of death: an anthropological account*. Edinburgh University Press.

Homan, R. (1991) *The ethics of social research*. London. Longman.

Hopper, A. (2000) 'Meeting the spiritual needs of patients through holistic practice', *European Journal of Palliative Care* **7**, 2.

Hornsby-Smith, M. and Whelan, C. (1994) 'Religious life and moral values', in C. Whelan (ed.), *Values and social change in Ireland*, 7–44. Dublin. Gill and Macmillan.

Howarth, G. (1993) 'Investigating deathwork: a personal account', in D. Clark (ed.), *The sociology of death*, 76–94. Oxford. Blackwell.

—— (1996) *Last rites: the work of the modern funeral director*. Amityville NY. Baywood Publishing.

—— (1998a) 'What's emotion got to do with it? Reflections on the personal in health research', *Annual Review of Health Social Sciences* **8**, 3–7.

——. (1998b) '"Just live for today". Living, caring, ageing and dying', *Ageing and Society* **18**, 673–89.

Hufford, D. (1982) *The terror that comes in the night: an experience-centred study of the supernatural*. University of Philadelphia Press.

Humphreys, J. (2002) 'Tragic choice of woman who most feared a failed suicide bid', *The Irish Times*, 2 February 2002.

Igoe, D., Keogh, F. and McNamara, C. (1997) 'A survey of Irish palliative care services', *Irish Journal of Medical Science* **166** (4), 206–11.

Illich, I. (1977) *Limits to medicine, medical nemesis: the expropriation of health*. London. Penguin Books.

Inglis, T. (1998) *Moral monopoly: the rise and fall of the Catholic Church in modern Ireland*. University College Dublin Press.

Irish Association of Palliative Care and the Irish Hospice Foundation (1996) *Position paper on the development of hospice and specialist palliative care services in Ireland*. Dublin.

Jalland, P. (1999) 'Victorian death and its decline 1850–1918', in P. Jupp and C. Gittings (eds), *Death in England: an illustrated history*, 230–55. Manchester University Press.

James, N. and Field, D. (1992) 'The routinization of hospice: charisma and bureaucratization', *Social Science and Medicine* **34** (12), 1363–75.

Jarrett, N., Payne, S., Turner, P. and Hiller, R. (1999) '"Someone to talk to" and "pain control": what people expect from a specialist palliative care team', *Palliative Medicine* **13**, 139–44.

Jenks, C. (1990) *What is Postmodernism*? London. Art and Design.

Kalish, R. and Reynolds, D. (1981) *Death and ethnicity: a psychocultural study*. Farmingdale NY. Baywood.

Kastenbaum, R. (1985) 'Do we die in stages?', in N. Datan and L. Ginsberg (eds), *Life span developmental psychology: normative life crises*, New York. Academic Press.

Kearney, M. (1992) 'Palliative medicine: just another speciality', *Palliative Medicine* **6**, 39–46.

—— (1996) *Mortally wounded: stories of soul pain, death and healing*. Dublin. Marino Books.

—— (2000) *A place of healing: working with suffering in living and dying*. Oxford

University Press.

Keegan, O. and van Doorslaer, O. (2001) *Contemporary Irish attitudes towards death, dying and bereavement*. Dublin. Health Services Research Centre, Royal College of Surgeons.

Keegan, O., McGee, H., Brady, T., Hogan, M., O'Brien, S. and O'Siorain, L. (1999) *Care for the dying—experiences and challenges: a study of quality of health service care during the last year of life of patients at St James's Hospital, Dublin, from their relatives' perspective*. Dublin. Irish Hospice Foundation.

Kellehear, A. (1989) 'Ethics and social research', in J. Perry (ed.), *Doing fieldwork: eight personal accounts of social research*. Geelong. Deakin University Press.

—— (1990) *Dying of cancer: the final year of life*. London. Harwood Academic Publishers.

—— (1998) 'Ethical issues for the qualitative researcher: some critical reflections', *Annual Review of Health Social Sciences* **8**, 14–17.

—— (2000a) *Experiences near death*. (First published 1996, New York, Oxford University Press.) Bridgewater NJ. Replica Books.

—— (2000b) 'Spirituality and palliative care: a model of needs', *Palliative Medicine* **14**, 149–55.

—— (2001) 'A good death', in G. Howarth and O. Leaman, *Encyclopedia of death and dying*, 209–10. London. Routledge.

—— (2002) 'Spiritual care in palliative care: whose job is it?', in B. Rumbold (ed.), *Spirituality and palliative care: social and pastoral perspectives*, 166–77. Victoria. Oxford University Press.

Kelner, M. J. and Bourgeault, C. (1993) 'Patient control over dying; response of health care professionals', *Social Science and Medicine* **36** (6), 757–65.

King, U. (1999) 'Spirituality, ageing and gender', in A. Jewell (ed.), *Spirituality and ageing*, 79–98. London. Jessica Kingsley.

Klass, D. (1981) 'Elisabeth Kübler-Ross and the tradition of the private sphere: an analysis of symbols', *Omega* **12** (3), 242–67.

—— Silverman, P. and Nickman, S. (eds) (1996) *Continuing bonds: new understandings of grief.* Bristol PA and London. Taylor and Francis.

Kübler-Ross, E. (1970) *On death and dying*. London. Tavistock.

Kvale, S. (1996) *InterViews: an introduction to qualitative research interviewing*. Thousand Oaks CA. Sage.

Larkin, P. (1999) 'The lived experience of Irish palliative care nurses', *International Journal of Palliative Nursing* **4** (3), 120–6.

Lawlor, B., Radic, A., Bruce, I., Swanwick, G. R. J., O'Kelly, F., O'Doherty, M., Walsh, J. B and Coakley, D. (1994) 'Prevalence of mental illness in an elderly community dwelling population using AGECAT', *Irish Journal of Psychological Medicine* **11** (4), 157–9.

Lawton, J. (2000) *The dying process: patients' experiences of palliative care*. London. Routledge.

Layder, D. (1993) *New strategies in social research*. Cambridge. Polity Press.

Lefebvre, H. (1991) *The production of space* (English translation). Oxford. Blackwell. Translated by Donald Nicholson-Smith.

Lofland, L. (1978) *The craft of dying: the modern face of death*. Beverly Hills. Sage.

Lundahl, C. (1982) *A collection of near-death research findings*. Chicago. Nelson-Hall Publishers.

Lunt, B. (1985) 'Terminal cancer care services: recent changes in regional inequalities in Great Britain', *Social Science and Medicine* **20** (7), 753–9.

Lyon, D. (2000) *Jesus in Disneyland: religion in postmodern times*. Cambridge. Polity Press.

Lysaght, P. (1995) 'Visible death: attitudes to the dying in Ireland', *Marvels and Tales* **9**, 27–60.

—— (1996) *The Banshee: the Irish supernatural death messenger*. Dublin. O'Brien Press.

—— (2001) 'The Banshee', in G. Howarth and O. Leaman, *Encyclopedia of death and dying*, 48–9. London. Routledge.

McDonnell, M. (1989) 'Patients' perception of care at Our Lady's Hospice, Dublin', *Palliative Care* **5**, 47–53.

McFarlane, A. and Kelleher, C. (2002) 'Concepts of illness causation and attitudes to health care among older people in the Republic of Ireland', *Social Science and Medicine* **54**, 1389–400.

McGowen, R. (1994) 'Power and humanity, or Foucault among the historians', in C. Jones and R. Porter (eds), *Reassessing Foucault*, 91–112. London. Routledge.

McNamara, B., Waddell, C. and Colvin, M. (1994) 'The institutionalization of the "good death"', *Social Science and Medicine* **39** (11), 1501–8.

—— (1995) 'Threats to the good death: the cultural context of stress and coping among hospice nurses', *Sociology of Health and Illness* **17** (2), 222–44.

McQuillan, R., Finlay, I., Roberts, D., Branch, C. and Spencer, M. G. (1996) 'The provision of a palliative care service in a teaching hospital and subsequent evaluation of that service', *Palliative Medicine* **10**, 231–9.

McSherry, W. (2001) 'Spiritual crisis? Call a nurse', in H. Orchard (ed.), *Spirituality in health care contexts*, 28–42. London. Jessica Kingsley Publishers.

Mak, J. M. (1992) 'Psychological responses to dying and death', *Senior Nurse* **1** (3), 48–51.

—— and Clinton, M. (1999) 'Promoting a good death: an agenda for outcomes research—a review of the literature', *Nursing Ethics* **6** (2), 97–106.

Materstvedt, L.J., Clark, D., Ellershaw, J., Førde, R., Boeck Gravgaard, A.M, Müller-Busch, H.C., Pota, I., Sales, J. and Rapin, C.H. (2003) 'Euthanasia and physician-assisted suicide: a view from the EAPC Ethics Task Force', *Palliative Medicine* **17**, 97–101.

Maxwell, E. (2001) 'Apostolic religious life in Ireland', in M. Breen (ed.), *A fire in the forest: religious life in Ireland*, 57–72. Dublin. Veritas Publications.

May, C. (1991) 'Affective neutrality and involvement in nurse–patient relationships: perceptions of appropriate behaviour among nurses in acute medical and surgical wards', *Journal of Advanced Nursing* **16**, 552–8.

May, J., Ellis-Hill, C. and Payne, S. (2001) 'Gatekeeping and legitimization; how informal carers' relationship with health care workers is revealed in their everyday interactions', *Journal of Advanced Nursing* **36** (3), 364–75.

Mead, G. H. (1934) *Mind, self and society*. University of Chicago Press.

Mennell, S. (1992) *Nobert Elias: an introduction*. Oxford. Blackwell Publishers.

—— (1996) *All manner of food: eating and taste in England and France from the Middle Ages to the present* (2nd edn). Illinois. Illini Books Edition.

Moane, G. (1996) 'Legacies of colonialism for Irish women', *Irish Journal of Feminist Studies* **1** (1), 100–18.

Morgan, P. (1999) 'Of worms and war', in P. Jupp and C. Gittings (eds), *Death in England: an illustrated history*, 119–48. Manchester University Press.

Morse, J. (2002) 'Qualitative health research: challenges for the 21st century', *Qualitative Health Research* **12** (1), 116–29.

Mount, B., MacDonald, N., Bruera, E. and Dudgeon, D. J. (1995) 'Ethical issues in palliative care research revisited', *Palliative Medicine* **9**, 165–6.

Murphy, E. and Dingwall, R. (2001) 'The ethics of ethnography', in P. Atkinson, A. Coffey, C. Delamont, J. Lofland and L. Lofland (eds), *Handbook of ethnography*, 175–203. London. Sage Publications.

Murray, M. and McMillan, C. (1993) 'Health beliefs, locus of control, emotional control and women's cancer screening behaviour', *British Journal of Clinical Psychology* **32**, 87–100.

Myers, K. (2003) 'An Irishman's Diary', *The Irish Times*, 20 March 2003.

—— (2004) 'An Irishman's Diary', *The Irish Times*, 22 June 2004.

Nandy, A. (1983) *The intimate enemy: loss and recovery of self under colonialism*. Delhi. Oxford University Press.

Narayanasamy, A. (1999) 'A review of spirituality as applied to nursing', International *Journal of Nursing Studies* **36**, 117–25.

NCH-SPCS (1996) *Palliative care services in the hospital setting*. Occasional Paper 10. London. National Council for Hospice and Specialist Palliative Care Services.

Nettleton, S. (1995) *The sociology of health and illness*. Cambridge. Polity Press.

Newman, C. (2000) 'Clergy disapprove of eulogies at funerals', *The Irish Times*, 30 March 2000.

Nimocks, M. J., Webb, J. and Connell, J. R. (1987) 'Communication and the terminally ill: a theoretical model', *Death Studies* **11**, 323–44.

Nocon, A. and Pearson, M. (2000) 'The roles of friends and neighbours in providing support for older people', *Ageing and Society* **20**, 341–67.

Noone, I., Crowe, M., Pillay, I. and O'Keeffe, S.T. (2000) 'Telling the truth about cancer: view of elderly patients and their relatives', *Irish Medical Journal* **93** (4), 104–5.

Novak, D., Plumer, R., Smith, R., Ochitill, H., Morrow, G. and Bennett, J. (1979) 'Changes to physicians' attitudes toward telling the cancer patient', *Journal of the American Medical Association* **241**, 897–900.

O'Boyle, C. and Waldron, D. (1997) 'Quality of life issues in palliative medicine', *Journal of Neurology* **244**, Supplement 4, S18–S25.

O'Brien, B. (2001) 'Dutch euthanasia is hardly death with dignity', *The Irish Times*, 14 April 2001.

O'Brien, T. (1995) 'Editorial', *Palliative Care Today* (Irish Supplement) **1**, 1–2.

Ó Donnabháin, B. (2000) 'An appalling vista? The Celts and the archaeology of later prehistoric Ireland', in A. Desmond, G. Johnson, M. McCarthy, J. Sheehan and E. Shee-Twohig (eds), *New agendas in Irish prehistory: papers in commemoration of Liz Anderson*, 189–96. Bray. Wordwell.

O'Donoghue, M. (1999) *Anam Cara: spiritual wisdom from the Celtic world*. New York. Bantam Books.

OECD (1997) *Economic surveys 1996–1997*. Paris. OECD.

Oken, D. (1961) 'What to tell cancer patients: a study of medical attitudes', *Journal of the American Medical Association* **175**, 1120–8.

O'Loughlin, T. (2000) *Journeys on the edge: the Celtic tradition*. London. Darton, Longman and Todd.

Olsen, K., Morse, J., Smith, J., Mayan, M. and Hammond, D. (2001) 'Linking trajectories of illness and dying', *Omega* **42** (4), 293–308.

Orchard, H. (2001) 'Being there? Presence and absence in spiritual care delivery', in H. Orchard (ed.), *Spirituality in health care contexts*, 97–123. London. Jessica

Kingsley Publishers.

O'Regan, E. (2001) 'Euthanasia must remain illegal, insist care experts', *The Irish Times*, 20 April 2001.

O'Shea, E. (2000) *The costs for caring for people with dementia and related cognitive impairments*. Report no. 60. Dublin. National Council on Ageing and Older People.

Osis, K. and Haraldsson, E. (1977) 'Deathbed observations by physicians and nurses: a cross-cultural survey', *Journal of the American Society for Psychical Research* **71** (3), 237–59.

O'Suilleabháin, S. (1967) *Irish wake amusements*. Cork. Mercier Press.

Papowitz, L. (1986) 'Lifedeathlife', *American Journal of Nursing* (April 1986), 416–21.

Patton, M. Q. (1990) *Qualitative evaluation and research methods* (2nd edn). Newbury Park CA. Sage. (1st edn 1980.)

Payne, S. (1997) 'Selecting an approach and design in qualitative research', *Palliative Medicine* **11**, 249–52.

Payne, S. A. and Langley-Evans, A. (1996) 'Perceptions of a "good" death: a comparative study of the views of hospice staff and patients', *Palliative Medicine* **10**, 307–12.

Pill, R. and Stott, N. (1982) 'Concepts of illness causation and responsibility, some preliminary data from a sample of working class mothers', *Social Science and Medicine* **16** (1), 43–52.

Porter, S. (1998) *Social theory and nursing practice*. Basingstoke. Macmillan.

Prior, L. (1989) *The social organisation of death*. Basingstoke. Macmillan.

Raban, J. (1990) *Hunting Mister Heartbreak*. London. Vintage Books.

Rae, S. and Smyth, S. (2002) 'Wife arranged her own death over internet', *Evening Herald*, 31 January 2002.

Randall, F. and Downie, R. S. (1996) *Palliative care ethics: a good companion*. Oxford University Press.

Raynes, N., Leach, J., Rawlings, B. and Bryson, R. (2000) 'Palliative care services:

views of terminally ill patients', *Palliative Medicine* **14**, 159–60.

Rees, W. D. (1971) 'The hallucinations of widowhood', *British Medical Journal* **2** (October), 37–41.

Reilly, J. (2002) 'Final exit opens up right-to-die inquiry', *Sunday Independent*, 3 February 2002.

Report of the National Advisory Committee on Palliative Care (2001) Department of Health and Children, Dublin.

Richards, M. A., Corner, J. and Clark, D. (1998) 'Developing a research culture for palliative care', *Palliative Medicine* **12**, 399–403.

Robinson, T. (1996) *Setting foot on the shores of Connemara and other writings*. Dublin. The Lilliput Press.

Rock, P. (2001) 'Symbolic interactionism and ethnography', in P. Atkinson, A. Coffey, C. Delamont, J. Lofland and L. Lofland (eds), *Handbook of ethnography*, 375–98. London. Sage Publications.

Rosenthal, C., Marshall, V. W., Macpherson, A. S.and French, S. E. (1980) *Nurses, patients and families*. London. Croom-Helm.

Ross, L. (1997) 'The nurse's role in assessing and responding to patients' spiritual needs', *International Journal of Palliative Nursing* **3** (1), 37–41.

Roy, D. (1987) 'The spiritual need of the dying' [Editorial], *Journal of Palliative Care* **2**, 2.

—— (1999) 'Why we need poets in palliative care' [Editorial], *Journal of Palliative Care* **15** (3), 3–5.

Rumbold, B. (2002) 'From religion to spirituality', in B. Rumbold (ed.), *Spirituality and palliative care: social and pastoral perspectives*, 5–21.Victoria. Oxford University Press.

Sandelowski, M. (2002) 'Reembodying qualitative inquiry', *Qualitative Health Research* **12** (1), 104–15.

Saunders, C. (1965) 'Watch with me', *Nursing Times* (26 Nov. 1965), 1–3.

—— (1976) 'Care of the dying', *Nursing Times* **72** (26), 3–24.

—— (1988) 'Spiritual pain', *Hospital Chaplain* (March 1988), 3–7.

—— (2003) 'Editorial: From the UK', *Palliative Medicine* **17**, 101–3.

—— and Kastenbaum, R. (eds) (1997) *Hospice care on the international scene*. New York. Springer Publishing Company.

Schoenbeck, S. (1993) 'Exploring the mystery of near-death experiences', *American Journal of Nursing* (May 1993), 43–6.

Seale, C. (1990) *The quality of qualitative research*. London. Sage.

—— (1998) *Constructing death: the sociology of dying and bereavement*. Cambridge University Press.

—— Addington-Hall, J. and McCarthy, M. (1997) 'Awareness of dying: prevalence, causes and consequences', *Social Science and Medicine* **45** (3), 477–84.

Sepúlveda, C., Marlin, A., Yoshida, T. and Ullrich, A. (2002) 'Palliative care: the World Health Organisation's global perspective', *Journal of Pain and Symptom Management* **24**, 91–6.

Seymour, J. (1999) 'Revisiting medicalisation and "natural" death', *Social Science and Medicine* **40**, 691–704.

Seymour, J. E. and Ingleton, C. (1999) 'Ethical issues in qualitative research at the end of life', *International Journal of Palliative Nursing* **5** (2), 65–73.

Sheehy, N. (1994) 'Death ritual as a cultural form', *The Irish Journal of Psychology* **15** (2 & 3), 494–507.

Shneidman, E. S. (1973) *Deaths of man*. Bath. Pitman.

Small, N. (1993) *Aids: the challenge*. Aldeshot. Avebury.

—— (1997) 'Death and difference', in D. Field, J. Hockey and N. Small, *Death, gender and ethnicity*, 202–21. London. Routledge.

—— (1998) 'Spirituality and hospice care', in M. Cobb and V. Robshaw (eds), *The spiritual challenge of health care*, 167–82. Edinburgh. Churchill Livingstone.

—— (2003) 'The changing National Health Service, user involvement and palliative care', in B. Munroe and D. Oliviere (eds), *Patient participation in palliative care: a voice for the voiceless*, 9–22. Oxford University Press.

Smith, D. C. and Maher, M. F. (1993) 'Achieving a healthy death: the dying person's attitudinal contributions', *Hospice Journal* **9**, 21–32.

Smyth, A. (ed.) (1992) *The Abortion Papers*. Dublin. Attic Press.

Sodestrom, K. and Martinson, I. (1987) 'Patient's spiritual coping strategies: a study of nurse and patient perspectives', *Oncology Nursing Forum* **14** (2), 41–6.

Sontag, S. (1989) *Aids and its metaphors*. London. Allan Lane.

Speck, P. (1998) 'The meaning of spirituality in illness', in M. Cobb and V. Robshaw (eds), *The spiritual challenge of health care*, 21–33. Edinburgh. Churchill Livingstone.

Spillar, J. A. and Alexander, D. A. (1993) 'Domiciliary care: a comparison of the views of terminally ill patients and their caregivers', *Palliative Medicine* **7**, 109–15.

Stanworth, R. (1997) 'Spirituality, language and depth of reality', *International Journal of Palliative Nursing* **3** (1), 19–22.

Stark, R. (1999) 'Secularization, R. I. P.', *Sociology of Religion* **60** (3), 249–73.

Stegnar, W. (1992) *Angle of repose* (first published 1971). New York. Penguin.

Steinhauser, K., Clipp, E., McNeilly, N., Christakis, N., McIntyre, L. and Tulsky, A. (2000) 'In search of a "good death": observations of patients, families and providers', *Annals of Internal Medicine* **132** (10), 825–32.

Storkey, M. (1993) *London's ethnic minorities: one city, many communities*. London Research Centre.

Surbone, A. (1992) 'Truth telling to the patient', *Journal of the American Medical Association* **268**, 1661–2.

Symonds, J. A. (1836) 'Signs of approaching death', in R. Todd (ed.), *The cyclopaedia of anatomy and physiology*, 798–803. London. Sherwood, Gilbert and Piper.

Szabo, S. (1996) 'The World Health Organisation quality of life assessment instrument', in B. Spiker (ed.), *Quality of life and pharmacoeconomics in clinical trials* (2nd edn), Philadelphia. Lippincott-Raven.

Taylor, H. (1983) *The hospice movement in Britain: its role and its functions*. London. Centre for Policy on Ageing.

Taylor, L. (1989) 'Bas in Eirinn: cultural constructions of death in Ireland', *Anthropological Quarterly* **62**, 175–87.

—— (1995) *Occasions of faith*. Dublin. Lilliput Press.

Tiernan, E., O'Connor, M., O'Siorain, L. and Kearney, M. (2002) 'A prospective study of preferred versus actual place of death among patients to a palliative care home-care service', *Irish Medical Journal* **95** (8), 232–5.

Townsend, J. (1993) 'Terminal cancer patients and patients' preference for place of death: a prospective study', *British Medical Journal* **301**, 415–17.

Van Doorslaer, O. and McQuillan, R. (2006) *The Travelling Community and the Specialist Palliative Care Services in the Eastern Region Health Authority*, Dublin. Irish Hospice Foundation.

Voltz, R., Akabayashi, A., Reese, C., Ohi, G. and Sass, H. M. (1997) 'Organisation and patients' perception of palliative care: a cross-cultural comparison', *Palliative Medicine* **11**, 351–7.

Walsh, D. (2001) 'Doing ethnography', in C. Seale (ed.), *Researching society and culture* (2nd edn), 271–94. London. Sage.

Walter, T. (1990) *Funerals and how to improve them*. London. Hodder and Stoughton.

—— (1994) *The revival of death*. London. Routledge.

—— (1997) 'The ideology and organisation of spiritual care: three approaches', *Palliative Medicine* **11**, 21–30.

—— (2002) 'Spirituality in palliative care: opportunity or burden?', *Palliative Medicine* **16**, 133–9.

Wasson, K. and George, R. (2001) 'Specialist palliative care for non-cancer patients: the ethical arguments', in J. Addington-Hall and A. Higginson (eds), *Palliative care for non-cancer patients*, 137–52. Oxford University Press.

Weisman, A. D. (1972) *On death and denying: a psychiatric study of terminality*. New York. Behavioural Publications.

—— (1974) *The realisation of death: a guide for psychological autopsy*. New York. Jason Aronson.

—— (1988) 'Appropriate death and the hospice program', *Hospice Journal* **4**, 65–77.

Weller, P. (ed.) (1997) *Religions in the UK: a multi-faith directory*. Derby. University of Derby and The Inter Faith Network.

WHO (1990) *Pain relief and palliative care*. Technical Report Series 804. Geneva. World Health Organisation.

Wilkes, E. (1980) *Terminal care: report of a working party*. London. HMSO.

Williams, G. and Popay, J. (1994) 'Lay knowledge and the privilege of experience', in J. Gabe, D. Kelleher and G. Williams (eds), *Challenging medicine*, 118–39. London. Routledge.

Williamson, R. (1990) *A Protestant legacy: attitudes to death and illness among older Aberdonians*. Oxford University Press.

Witoszek, N. and Sheeran, P. (1994) *The Irish funerary tradition*. Research Report 4. Social Science Research Centre, University College Galway.

Wren, M. A. (2003) *An unhealthy state: an anatomy of a sick society*. Dublin. New Island.

Wright, M. (2001) 'Chaplaincy in hospice and hospital: findings for a survey in England and Wales', *Palliative Medicine* **15**, 229–42.

Young, M. and Cullen, L. (1996) *A good death: conversations with East Londoners*. London. Routledge.

Zaleski, C. (1987) *Otherworld journeys: accounts of near-death experience in medieval and modern times*. New York. Oxford University Press.

INDEX

Una MacConville

Dr. Una MacConville is a Visiting Fellow at the Centre for Death and Society in the Department of Social and Policy Sciences, and Lecturer and Module Leader for the Foundation Degree in Funeral Services (Religion, Spirituality and Secularisation) at the University of Bath in the United Kingdom. Dr. MacConville holds a Ph.D. in Sociology from the Department of Social and Policy Sciences at the University of Bath.